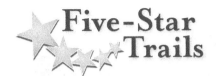

Five-Star Trails

Chattanooga

40 Spectacular Hikes in and around the Scenic City

2ND EDITION

T0125561

JOHNNY MOLLOY

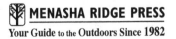

MENASHA RIDGE PRESS
Your Guide to the Outdoors Since 1982

Five-Star Trails: Chattanooga

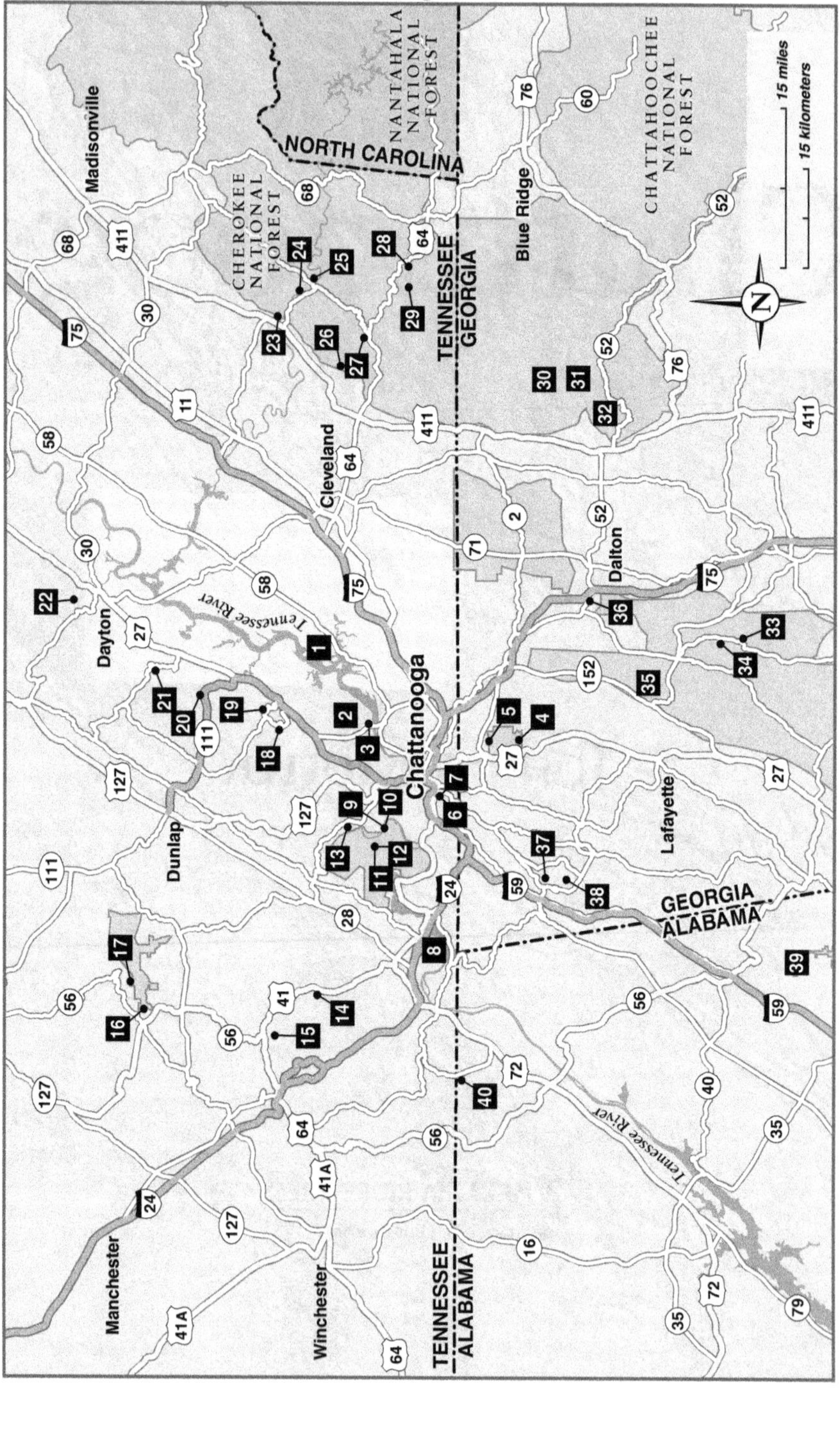

Overview Map Key

Library of Congress Cataloging-in-Publication Data

Names: Molloy, Johnny, 1961– author.
Title: Five-star trails : Chattanooga : 40 spectacular hikes near the scenic city / Johnny Molloy.
Description: Second Edition. | Birmingham : Menasha Ridge Press, 2020. | Series: Five-star trails |
    First edition published 2013.
Identifiers: LCCN 2020025992 (print) | LCCN 2020025993 (ebook) | ISBN 9781634043052 (paperback) |
    ISBN 9781634043069 (ebook)
Subjects: LCSH: Hiking—Tennessee—Chattanooga—Guidebooks. | Trails—Tennessee—Chattanooga—
    Guidebooks. | Chattanooga (Tenn.)—Guidebooks.
Classification: LCC GV199.42.T22 C426 2020 (print) | LCC GV199.42.T22 (ebook) |
    DDC 796.5109768/82—dc23
LC record available at https://lccn.loc.gov/2020025992
LC ebook record available at https://lccn.loc.gov/2020025993

 MENASHA RIDGE PRESS
An imprint of AdventureKEEN
2204 First Ave. S., Ste. 102
Birmingham, AL 35233
800-678-7006, fax 877-374-9016

Visit menasharidge.com for a complete listing of our books and for ordering information. Contact us at our
website, at facebook.com/menasharidge, or at twitter.com/menasharidge with questions or comments. To find
out more about who we are and what we're doing, visit blog.menasharidge.com.

Table of Contents

Tennessee Appalachians 134

North Georgia and Northeast Alabama 172

Appendixes

Dedication

This book is for all the residents of greater Chattanooga. You are blessed with abundant beauty.

 # Acknowledgments

Thanks to all the people who have constructed, maintained, and advocated trails and hiking in Chattanooga and beyond.

Preface

WELCOME TO THE SECOND EDITION OF THIS GUIDE. New hikes have been added, and the book has been completely updated. Chattanooga is an outdoorsy town. Consistently rated in surveys as among the best places to live for outdoors enthusiasts, Chattanooga is located within easy reach of a wide array of paddling, camping, and especially hiking destinations. The city's expanding greenways and parks programs have garnered national attention.

The natural setting has been there all along.

Geographically speaking, Chattanooga couldn't be better situated for offering a variety of terrain and trails on which to trek. Centered on the banks of the mighty Tennessee River, just before that waterway enters the Grand Canyon of the Tennessee River, Chattanooga is flanked to the east by the lofty Southern Appalachian Mountains and to the west by the rugged Cumberland Plateau. Historic and noteworthy peaks rise within sight of town.

This nexus of mountain and river is partially responsible for Chattanooga's extensive parklands. The town was an important place of contention between the Union and the Confederacy during the Civil War. The places where they clashed have been preserved as parks to commemorate the history of that time. Today, trails lace these former battlefields.

The Cumberland Plateau, the Tennessee River Valley, and the Southern Appalachians ignore state boundaries and present hiking opportunities not only in Tennessee but also in Georgia and Alabama. The melding of these three physiographic provinces among these three states sets the stage for hikers. And there are many destinations for hikers to ramble on this varied stage. The Cumberland Plateau rises just to the west of Chattanooga. The Plateau, as it is known in these parts, offers distinct terrain with correspondingly unusual hiking experiences. Here, water-carved gorges slice through an elevated tableland, exposing rock walls and creating rock houses, stone arches, sheer bluffs, and other geological features that complement the green expanse of the Southern Appalachians.

Cumberland Plateau hiking destinations include Savage Gulf State Natural Area, Grundy Forest, and the series of steep and magnificent gorges flowing off the east side of the Plateau into the Tennessee River. The most famous gorge may be Laurel Snow, through which Richland Creek carves its canyon from the Plateau

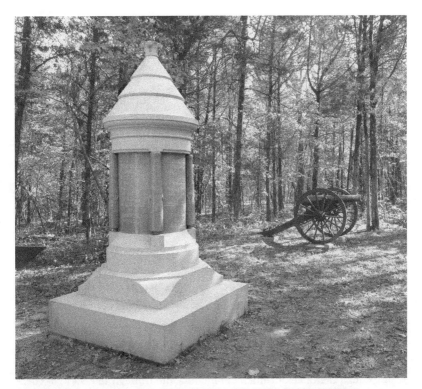

MEMORIALS AND CANNON EMPLACEMENTS TELL THE STORY OF CHICKAMAUGA BATTLEFIELD. (SEE HIKE 5, PAGE 40)

to the lowlands. Lesser-known yet equally scenic places like Possum Creek Gorge also feature the Cumberland Trail winding its way north. Don't forget DeSoto State Park in Alabama, too, with its share of geological features and waterfalls.

To the east rise the magnificent Appalachians. Here, mountain peaks soar for the sky, while rushing streams race for the lowlands. Large and varied tree species carpet rugged ridges, colorful wildflowers thrive in the streamside flats, and bears roam the roughs. In our Southern Highlands, explorers can hike through resplendent wilderness along chilly, trout-filled streams; soak in upland vistas; and escape to the back of beyond. Hike to the falls astride Gee Creek, or along the banks of the ridge-rimmed Big Lost Creek, or grab a view from piney outcrops atop Fort Mountain.

The Tennessee Valley is no flatland itself. Chattanooga can be a hilly town. And with citizens interested in hiking, it is only natural that trails and greenways aplenty have been created in the greater metropolitan area—making moving your feet even more convenient. Trekking in the Tennessee Valley adds one more spice to the entrée of offerings in addition to the Southern Appalachians and the Cumberland Plateau.

So hiking in Chattanooga can mean a ramble through the backcountry of the Big Frog Wilderness, a trek to a natural bridge on the Cumberland Plateau, or a quick escape on a greenway near your house. It all depends on your mood, company, and desires. Therefore, not only is the "where to hike" component covered in this book, so is "what type of hike." As to when: You can hike year-round in Chattanooga—whether it be in the heat of summer, when you can escape to the high country, or in the chill of winter, when the trails of the Tennessee River Valley can still be enjoyed no matter the temperature.

That is where this book comes into play. The variety of hikes contained within its pages reflects the variety of opportunities in this region. I sought to include day hikes covering routes of multiple lengths, ranging from easy to difficult. Trail configurations are diverse as well, including out-and-back hikes, loops, balloon loops, and even double loops. Hike settings vary from the city of Chattanooga to secluded gorges to distant mountaintops.

The routes befit a range of athletic prowess and hiking experience. Simply scan through the table of contents, randomly flip through the book, or check out the recommended hikes list. Find your hike, get out there, and enjoy it. And bring a friend too. Enjoying nature in the company of another is a great way to enhance your relationship as well as escape from your smartphone, television, and other electronic chains that bind us to the daily grind.

Recommended Hikes

Best for Dogs

Best for Geology

Best for Human History

Best for Kids

Best for Scenery

Best for Seclusion

Best for Views

Best for Waterfalls

Best for Water Lovers

Best for Wildflowers

Best for Wildlife

FOSTER FALLS CHARGES 60 FEET OVER A STONE LIP INTO A MASSIVE PLUNGE POOL. (SEE HIKE 14, PAGE 88)

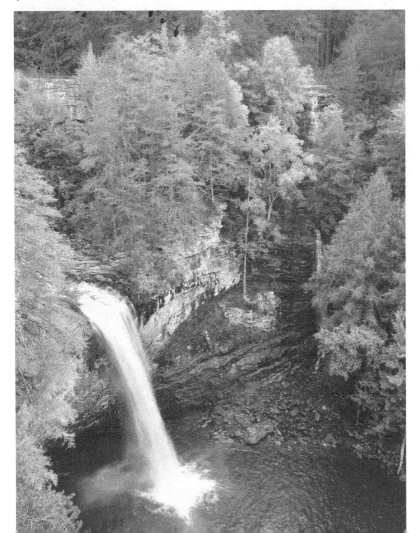

Map Legend

←→ ➡	═══════════	‑ ‑ ‑ ‑ ‑ ‑ ‑ ‑ ‑
Directional arrows	Featured trail	Alternate trail
▬▬▬▬▬▬	════╤════	═══════════
Freeway	Highway with bridge	Minor road
▪▪▪▪▪▪▪▪▪▪▪	∙∙∙∙∙∙∙∙∙∙∙	═ ═ ═ ═ ═ ═
Boardwalk	Stairs	Unpaved road
┼┼┼┼┼┼┼┼┼	•—•—•—•	▬ ∙ ▬ ∙ ▬
Railroad	Power line	Border
▭	◞	⌇
Park/forest	Water body	River/creek/ intermittent stream wash

♨ Amphitheater	✳ Garden	⛱ Picnic area
⌐ Bench	● General point of interest	🏠 Picnic shelter
⛵ Boat launch	🏌 Golf course	▲ Primitive camping
✕ Bridge	🧍 Lookout tower	⊪ Scenic view
⌂ Cabin	⚓ Marina	○ Spring
▲ Camping	✕ Mine/quarry	🧍 Trailhead
𝄞 Cascades	⚊ Monument	⬆ Viewing platform
⚏ Cemetery	△ Overlook	// Waterfall
⚲ Church	⌂ Park office	⌇ Wetland
╱ Dam	🅿 Parking	
⦀ Food service	▲ Peak	

Introduction

About This Book

FIVE-STAR TRAILS: CHATTANOOGA details 40 great hikes in Chattanooga and the immediate region. It presents the reader with an array of treks that reflect the magnificence of the area, ranging from the Cumberland Plateau to the Tennessee River Valley to the Southern Appalachians. Often referred to as the Scenic City, Chattanooga is a great jumping-off point for hikers, where immediate urban and suburban hikes can satiate scenery-hungry residents while the superlative beauty of the adjacent national and state parks is just a short drive away. All this adds up to a hiker's nirvana.

In fact, I firmly believe Chattanooga is one of the best outdoors towns in the United States. To our east and south we have large tracts of national forest, Tennessee's Cherokee National Forest, and Georgia's Chattahoochee National Forest. Hundreds of miles of trails lace these mountain lands. The Cherokee and Chattahoochee also offer camping, hunting, fishing, nature study, and more. The geologically fascinating Cumberland Plateau rises to the west; there you can hike your way past rushing rivers, deep gorges, wild waterfalls, and other rock features. Hikes in this book cover state parks and forests in all four cardinal directions, from the untamed splendor of Prentice Cooper State Forest rising to the west, to the deep gorge of Chickamauga Creek lying north, to view-laden Fort DeSoto in the south, to the Big Frog Wilderness in the east.

And Chattanooga's climate is ideal for hiking; we have four distinct and beautiful seasons. If you like winter, the mountains deliver a surprising amount of snow above 4,000 feet! Yet many mild days occur that are perfect for trail trekkers. The elevation and terrain variations make spring exciting too. Rebirth spreads from the lowlands to the high country, and wildflowers follow. Summer finds many of us escaping to cool waters and to refreshing mountaintops where heat-relieving breezes blow. During fall, Chattanooga's incredible variety of trees explode in their annual color display.

How do you get started? Peruse this book, pick out a hike, and strike out on the trail. The wide assortment of paths, distances, difficulties, and destinations will suit any hiker's mood and company. And try them all—the varied hikes will leave you appreciating the nature of greater Chattanooga more than you ever imagined. Enjoy!

Greater Chattanooga's Geographic Divisions

The hikes in this book are split into four geographic divisions. **Greater Chattanooga** covers hikes within the city limits and the metro area, encompassing both Tennessee and the northwest corner of Georgia. The hikes here include Chattanooga's abundant and expanding greenway system. Here you can make a quick escape for daily exercise or explore historic parks like Chattanooga & Chickamauga National Military Park. This section also includes nearby Prentice Cooper State Forest. Hike along the banks of the Tennessee River through its deep canyon, or explore one of the Tennessee Valley Authority's small wild areas such as Little Cedar Mountain.

Tennessee Cumberlands includes hikes on the Cumberland Plateau within the bounds of the Volunteer State and segments of the Cumberland Trail, Tennessee's master path slated to extend from Signal Mountain north to Cumberland Gap at the Kentucky state line. In this area, you can hike at scenic Savage Gulf State Natural Area, lesser-visited Rock Creek Gorge, or deep into the chasm created by North Chickamauga Creek.

The hikes of the **Tennessee Appalachians** section stretch from the historic trek on the Old Copper Road Trail to the glissading cascades of Benton Falls. Other wild treks take in the Big Frog Wilderness and Benton MacKaye Trail as it wanders along Big Lost Creek. Visit the lonely backwoods of Gee Creek or discover the Falls of the Scenic Spur.

North Georgia and Northeast Alabama comprises the Peach State's remote and unrefined Chattahoochee National Forest, select Georgia state parks, and the northeast corner of the Yellowhammer State. Grab a view of Keown Falls, or loop through The Pocket. The Chattahoochee offers superlative Southern Appalachian scenery and destinations, from wildernesses to waterfalls to overlooks. More highlights bring in area history and beauty from Russell Cave National Monument to the untamed Sitton Gulch. Altogether, the trail-laced geographic regions of greater Chattanooga create a mosaic of natural splendor that will please the most discriminating hiker.

How to Use This Guidebook

Overview Map, Map Key, and Map Legend

The overview map on page ii depicts the location of the primary trailhead for all 40 of the hikes described in this book. The numbers shown on the overview map pair with the map key on the facing page. Each hike's number remains with that hike throughout the book. Thus, if you spot an appealing hiking area on the overview map, you can flip through the book and find those hikes easily by their numbers at the top of each profile page. A legend identifying the map symbols used throughout the book appears on page xiv.

Trail Maps

In addition to the overview map, a detailed map of each hike's route appears with its profile. On this map, symbols indicate the trailhead, the complete route, significant features, facilities, and topographic landmarks such as creeks, overlooks, and peaks.

To produce the highly accurate maps in this book, I used a handheld GPS unit to gather data while hiking each route, then sent that data to the publisher's expert cartographers.

Elevation Profile

This diagram represents the rises and falls of the trail as viewed from the side, over the complete distance (in miles) of that trail. On the diagram's vertical axis, or height scale, the number of feet indicated between each tick mark lets you visualize the climb. To avoid making flat hikes look steep and steep hikes appear flat, varying height scales provide an accurate image of each hike's climbing difficulty. For example, one hike's scale might rise to 200 feet, while another goes to 2,000 feet.

The Hike Profile

Each profile opens with the hike's star ratings, GPS trailhead coordinates, and other key at-a-glance information—from the trail's distance and configuration to contacts for local information. Each profile also includes a map (see "Trail Maps," above). The main text for each profile includes four sections: Overview, Route Details, Nearby Attractions, and Directions (for driving to the trailhead area).

Star Ratings

Following is the explanation for the rating system of one to five stars in each of the five categories for each hike.

FOR SCENERY:

★ ★ ★ ★ ★	Unique, picturesque panoramas
★ ★ ★ ★	Diverse vistas
★ ★ ★	Pleasant views
★ ★	Unchanging landscape
★	Not selected for scenery

FOR TRAIL CONDITION:

★ ★ ★ ★ ★	Consistently well maintained
★ ★ ★ ★	Stable, with no surprises
★ ★ ★	Average terrain to negotiate
★ ★	Inconsistent, with good and poor areas
★	Rocky, overgrown, or often muddy

FOR CHILDREN:

★ ★ ★ ★ ★	Babes in strollers are welcome
★ ★ ★ ★	Fun for anyone past the toddler stage
★ ★ ★	Good for young hikers with proven stamina
★ ★	Not enjoyable for children
★	Not advisable for children

FOR DIFFICULTY:

★ ★ ★ ★ ★	Grueling
★ ★ ★ ★	Strenuous
★ ★ ★	Moderate (won't beat you up—but you'll know you've been hiking)
★ ★	Easy with patches of moderate
★	Good for a relaxing stroll

FOR SOLITUDE:

★ ★ ★ ★ ★	Positively tranquil
★ ★ ★ ★	Spurts of isolation
★ ★ ★	Moderately secluded
★ ★	Crowded on weekends and holidays
★	Steady stream of individuals and/or groups

GPS TRAILHEAD COORDINATES

As noted in "Trail Maps," above, I used a handheld GPS unit to obtain geographic data and sent the information to the publisher's cartographers. In the key information for each hike profile, I have provided the intersection of the latitude (north) and longitude (west) coordinates to orient you at the trailhead. In some cases, you can drive within viewing distance of a trailhead. Other hikes require a short walk to reach the trailhead from a parking area. Either way, the trailhead coordinates are given from the trail's actual head—its point of origin.

You will also note that this guidebook uses the degree–decimal minute format for presenting the GPS coordinates. The latitude and longitude grid system is likely quite familiar to you, but here is a refresher, pertinent to visualizing the GPS coordinates: Imaginary lines of latitude—called parallels and approximately 69 miles apart from each other—run horizontally around the globe. Each parallel is indicated by degrees from the equator (established to be 0°): up to 90°N at the North Pole and down to 90°S at the South Pole.

Imaginary lines of longitude, called meridians, run perpendicular to latitude lines. Longitude lines are likewise indicated by degrees: starting from 0° at the Prime Meridian in Greenwich, England, they continue to the east and west until they meet 180° later at the International Date Line in the Pacific Ocean. At the equator, longitude lines also are approximately 69 miles apart, but that distance narrows as the meridians converge toward the North and South Poles.

To convert GPS coordinates given in degrees, minutes, and seconds to the degree–decimal minute format, the seconds are divided by 60. For more on GPS technology, visit usgs.gov.

DISTANCE & CONFIGURATION

Distance indicates the length of the hike from start to finish, either round-trip or one-way depending on the trail configuration. If the hike description includes options to shorten or extend the hike, those distances will also be factored here. **Configuration** defines the type of route—for example, an out-and-back (which takes you in and out the same way), a figure eight, a loop, or a balloon.

HIKING TIME

A general rule of thumb for the hiking times noted in this guidebook is 1.5 miles per hour. That pace typically allows time for taking photos, for dawdling and admiring views, and for alternating stretches of hills and descents. When deciding whether or not to follow a particular trail in this guidebook, consider your own pace, the weather, your general physical condition, and your energy level that day.

HIGHLIGHTS

This section lists features that draw hikers to the trail: waterfalls, historic sites, and the like.

ELEVATION

In each hike's key information, you'll see the elevation (in feet) at the trailhead and another figure for the peak height or low point on that route. The hike profile also includes an elevation diagram (see page 3).

ACCESS

Fees or permits required to hike the trail are detailed here—and noted if there are none. Trail-access hours are also shown here.

MAPS

Resources for maps, in addition to those in this guidebook, are listed here. (As previously noted, the publisher and I recommend that you carry more than one map—and that you consult those maps before heading out on the trail in order to resolve any confusion or discrepancy.)

ENJOY VIEWS LIKE THIS ON THE SOUTH CHICKAMAUGA BATTLEFIELD LOOP. (SEE HIKE 4, PAGE 35)

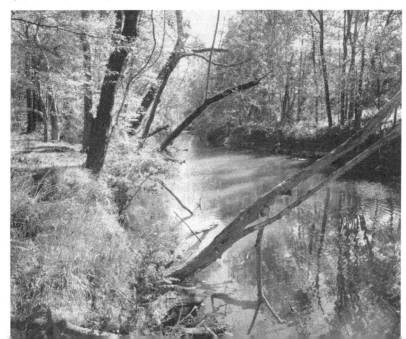

FACILITIES

This section alerts you to restrooms, phones, water, picnic tables, and other basics at or near the trailhead.

WHEELCHAIR ACCESS

Paved sections or other areas where one can safely use a wheelchair are noted here.

COMMENTS

Here you'll find assorted nuggets of information, such as whether or not dogs are allowed on the trails.

CONTACTS

Listed here are phone numbers and website addresses for checking trail conditions and gleaning other day-to-day information.

Overview, Route Details, Nearby Attractions, and Directions

These four elements provide the main text about the hike. "Overview" gives you a quick summary of what to expect on that trail; the "Route Details" guide you on the hike, start to finish; "Nearby Attractions" suggests appealing area sites, such as restaurants, museums, and other trails; and "Directions" will get you to the trailhead from a well-known road or highway.

Weather

Each of the four seasons distinctly lays its hands on Chattanooga. Summer can be fairly hot, but that is when hikers head for the mountains. Thunderstorms can pop up in the afternoons. If hiking in Chattanooga city limits during summer, I recommend going early in the morning or late in the evening. Hikers really hit the trails when fall's first northerly fronts sweep cool, clear air across the Scenic City and adjacent environs. Mountaintop vistas are best enjoyed during this time. Crisp mornings give way to warm afternoons. Fall is drier than summer and is the driest of all seasons. Winter can bring frigid subfreezing days and chilling rains—and snow in the high country. However, a brisk hiking pace will keep you warm. Each cold month has several days of mild weather. Spring will be more variable. A warm day can be followed by a cold one. Extensive spring rains bring regrowth, but also keep hikers indoors. But avid hikers will find more good hiking days than they will have time to hike in spring and every other season. To give you an idea of what weather to expect, the chart below details Chattanooga's monthly averages. Expect cooler temperatures on the Cumberland Plateau and the Southern Appalachians.

MONTH	HIGH	LOW	PRECIPITATION
January	50°F	31°F	4.9 inches
February	55°F	34°F	5.0 inches
March	64°F	41°F	5.0 inches
April	73°F	48°F	4.0 inches
May	80°F	57°F	4.1 inches
June	87°F	66°F	4.1 inches
July	90°F	70°F	4.9 inches
August	90°F	69°F	3.5 inches
September	83°F	62°F	4.0 inches
October	73°F	50°F	3.3 inches
November	62°F	40°F	5.0 inches
December	52°F	33°F	4.9 inches

Source: usclimatedata.com

Water

How much is enough? Well, one simple physiological fact should convince you to err on the side of excess when deciding how much water to pack: a hiker walking steadily in 90-degree heat needs approximately 10 quarts of fluid per day. That's 2.5 gallons. A good rule of thumb is to hydrate prior to your hike, carry (and drink) 6 ounces of water for every mile you plan to hike, and hydrate again after the hike. For most people, the pleasures of hiking make carrying water a relatively minor price to pay to remain safe and healthy. So pack more water than you anticipate needing, even for short hikes.

If you are tempted to drink "found water," do so with extreme caution. Many ponds and lakes encountered by hikers are fairly stagnant and taste terrible, plus they present inherent risks for thirsty trekkers. Giardia parasites contaminate many water sources and cause the dreaded intestinal ailment giardiasis, which can last for weeks after ingestion. For information, visit the Centers for Disease Control website at cdc.gov/parasites/giardia.

In any case, effective treatment is essential before using any water source found along the trail. Boiling water for 2–3 minutes is always a safe measure for camping, but day hikers can consider iodine tablets, approved chemical mixes, filtration units rated for giardia, and UV filtration. Some of these methods (e.g., filtration with an added carbon filter) remove bad tastes typical in stagnant water, while others add their own taste. Carry a means of purification to help in a pinch and if you realize you have underestimated your consumption needs.

Clothing

Weather, unexpected trail conditions, fatigue, extended hiking duration, and wrong turns can individually or collectively turn a great outing into a very uncomfortable one at best—and a life-threatening one at worst. Thus, proper attire plays a key role in staying comfortable and, sometimes, staying alive. Here are some helpful guidelines:

★ Choose silk, wool, or synthetics for maximum comfort in all of your hiking attire—from hats to socks and in-between. Cotton is fine if the weather remains dry and stable, but you won't be happy if it gets wet.

★ Always wear a hat, or at least tuck one into your day pack or hitch it to your belt. Hats offer all-weather sun and wind protection as well as warmth if it turns cold.

★ Be ready to layer up or down as the day progresses and the mercury rises or falls. Today's outdoor wear makes layering easy, with such designs as jackets that convert to vests and zip-off or button-up pant legs.

★ Wear hiking boots or sturdy hiking sandals with toe protection. Flip-flopping on a paved path in an urban botanical garden is one thing, but never hike a trail in open sandals or casual sneakers. Your bones and arches need support, and your skin needs protection.

★ Pair that footwear with good socks! If you prefer not to sheathe your feet when wearing hiking sandals, tuck the socks into your day pack; you may need them if the weather plummets or if you hit rocky turf and pebbles begin to irritate your feet. And, in an emergency, if you have lost your gloves, you can adapt the socks into mittens.

★ Don't leave rainwear behind, even if the day dawns clear and sunny. Tuck into your day pack, or tie around your waist, a jacket that is breathable and either water-resistant or waterproof. Investigate different choices at your local outdoors retailer. If you are a frequent hiker, ideally you'll have more than one rainwear weight, material, and style in your closet to protect you in all seasons in your regional climate and hiking microclimates.

Essential Gear

Today you can buy vests that have up to 20 pockets shaped and sized to carry everything from toothpicks to binoculars. Or, if you don't aspire to feel like a burro, you can neatly stow all of these items in your day pack or backpack. The following list showcases never-hike-without-them items:

★ *Water:* As emphasized more than once in this book, bring more than you think you will drink; depending on your destination, you may want to bring a water bottle and iodine or a filter for purifying water in the wilderness in case you run out.

★ *Map and high-quality compass:* Even if you know the terrain from previous hikes, don't leave home without these tools. If you are versed with a GPS bring that, too, but don't rely on it as your sole navigational tool—batteries can die.

★ *A pocketknife and/or multitool*

★ *A flashlight or headlamp with an extra bulb and batteries*

★ *Windproof matches and/or a lighter,* as well as a fire starter

★ *Extra food:* Trail mix, granola bars, or other high-energy foods

★ *Extra clothes:* Raingear, warm hat, gloves, and change of socks and shirt

★ *Whistle:* This little gadget will be your best friend in an emergency.

★ *Insect repellent:* When you want it, you really want it. Bring a small bottle with deet in it.

★ *Sunscreen:* Note the expiration date on the tube or bottle; it's usually embossed on the top.

★ *Today's handheld devices* have not only a phone that may help you contact help, but also built-in GPS that can help with orientation. However, do not call for help unless you are truly in need, and remember that smartphone batteries can die, though a cell battery pack helps. Additionally, you can use your smartphone to download park maps for reference. However, download maps at home rather than taking chances with reception in the hinterlands. And be sure your device is fully charged before your hike, so you'll have access to your maps for the duration of your hike.

First Aid Kit

Combined with the items above, those below may appear overwhelming for a day hike. But any paramedic will tell you that the items listed here, in alphabetical order, are just the basics. The reality of hiking is that you can be out for a week of backpacking and acquire only a mosquito bite—or you can hike for an hour, slip, and suffer a bleeding abrasion or broken bone. Fortunately, these items will collapse into a very small space, and convenient prepackaged kits are available at your pharmacy and on the internet.

Consider your intended terrain and the number of hikers in your party before you exclude any item listed below. A botanical garden stroll may not inspire you to carry a complete kit, but anything beyond that warrants precaution. When hiking alone, you should always be prepared for a medical need. And if you are a twosome or a group, one or more people in your party should be equipped with first aid material.

★ Ace bandages or Spenco joint wraps

★ Antibiotic ointment (Neosporin or the generic equivalent)

★ Athletic tape

★ Band-Aids

★ Benadryl or the generic equivalent diphenhydramine (in case of allergic reactions)

★ Blister kit (such as Moleskin/Spenco Second Skin)

★ Butterfly-closure bandages

★ Epinephrine in a prefilled syringe (for people known to have severe allergic reactions to such things as bee stings; usually by prescription only)

★ Gauze (one roll and a half dozen 4-x-4-inch pads)

★ Hydrogen peroxide or iodine

★ Ibuprofen or acetaminophen

General Safety

The following tips may have the familiar ring of your mother's voice as you take note of them:

★ *Always let someone know where you will be hiking* and how long you expect to be gone. It's a good idea to give that person a copy of your route, particularly if you are headed into any isolated area. Let that person know when you return.

★ *Always sign in and out of any trail registers provided.* Don't hesitate to comment on the trail condition if space is provided; that's your opportunity to alert others to any problems you encounter.

★ *Do not count on a cell phone for your safety.* Reception may be spotty or nonexistent on the trail, even on an urban walk embraced by towering trees.

★ *Always carry food and water,* even for a short hike.

★ *Stay on designated trails.* Even on the most clearly marked trails, there is usually a point where you have to stop and consider in which direction to head. If you become disoriented, don't panic. As soon as you think you may be off-track, stop, assess your current direction, and then retrace your steps to the point where you went astray. Using a map, a compass, a GPS, and this book, and keeping in mind what you have passed thus far, reorient yourself and trust your judgment on which way to continue. Also, see if your smartphone or handheld device has map capability and you can use it for orientation. If you become absolutely unsure of how to continue, return to your vehicle the way you came in. Should you become completely lost and have no idea how to return to the trailhead, remaining in place along the trail and waiting for help is most often the best option for adults and always the best option for children.

★ *Be especially careful when crossing streams.* Whether you are fording the stream or crossing on a log, make every step count. If you have any doubt about maintaining your balance on a log, ford the stream instead: use a trekking pole or stout stick for balance and face upstream as you cross. If a stream seems too deep to ford, turn back. Whatever is on the other side is not worth risking your life.

★ *Be careful at overlooks.* While these areas may provide spectacular views, they are potentially hazardous. Stay back from the edge of outcrops and be absolutely sure of your footing; a misstep can mean a nasty and possibly fatal fall.

★ *Standing dead trees and storm-damaged living trees* pose a real hazard to hikers. These trees may have loose or broken limbs that could fall at any time. While walking beneath trees, and when choosing a spot to rest or enjoy your snack, look up!

★ *Know the symptoms of hypothermia.* Shivering and forgetfulness are the two most common indicators of this stealthy killer. Hypothermia can occur at any elevation, even in the summer, especially when the hiker is wearing lightweight cotton clothing. If symptoms present themselves, get to shelter, hot liquids, and dry clothes ASAP.

★ *Ask questions.* National forest, state forest, and other park employees are there to help. It's a lot easier to ask advice beforehand, and it will help you avoid a mishap away from civilization when it's too late to amend an error.

★ *Most important of all, take along your brain.* A cool, calculating mind is the single-most important asset on the trail. Think before you act. Watch your step. Plan ahead. Avoiding accidents before they happen is the best way to ensure a rewarding and relaxing hike.

Animal, Insect, and Plant Hazards

Black Bears Though attacks by black bears are very rare, they have happened in the Southern Appalachians, even within the radius this guide covers. The sight or approach of a bear can give anyone a start. If you encounter a bear while hiking, remain calm and never run away. Make loud noises to scare off the bear and back away slowly. In primitive and remote areas, assume bears are present; in more developed sites, check on the current bear situation prior to hiking. Most encounters are food related, as bears have an exceptional sense of smell and not particularly discriminating tastes. While this is of greater concern to backpackers and campers, on a day hike, you may plan a lunchtime picnic or munch on an energy bar or other snack from time to time. So remain aware and alert.

SNAKES Rattlesnakes, cottonmouths, copperheads, and corals are among the most common venomous snakes in the United States, and hibernation season is typically October–April. In greater Chattanooga, you will possibly encounter the timber rattler or copperhead. However, the snakes you most likely will see while hiking will be nonvenomous. The best rule is to leave all snakes alone, give them a wide berth as you hike past, and make sure any hiking companions (including dogs) do the same.

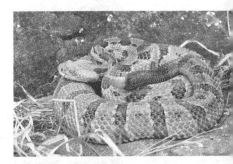

TIMBER RATTLESNAKE
Photographed by James DeBoer/Shutterstock

When hiking, stick to well-used trails and wear over-the-ankle boots and loose-fitting long pants. Rattlesnakes like to bask in the sun and won't bite unless threatened. Do not step or put your hands where you cannot see, and avoid wandering around in the dark. Step onto logs and rocks, never over them, and be especially careful when climbing rocks. Always avoid walking through dense brush or willow thickets. Copperheads are most often found along streams, also looking for a sunny spot atop a rock.

MOSQUITOES These little naggers are found more often in the city of Chattanooga but sparingly in the hillier Plateau and Southern Appalachians. Insect repellent and/or repellent-impregnated clothing are the only simple methods to ward off these pests. In some areas, mosquitoes are known to carry the West Nile virus, so all due caution should be taken to avoid their bites.

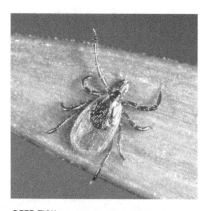

DEER TICK Photographed by Jim Gathany/Centers for Disease Control and Prevention (public domain)

TICKS Ticks are often found on brush and in tall grass, where they seem to be waiting to hitch a ride on a warm-blooded passerby. Adult ticks are most active April into May and again October into November. Among the varieties of ticks, the black-legged tick, commonly called the deer tick, is the primary carrier of Lyme disease. Wear light-colored clothing so that ticks can be spotted before they make it to the skin. And be sure to visually check your hair, back of neck, armpits, and socks at the end of the hike. During your post-hike shower, take a moment to do a more complete body check. For ticks that are already embedded, removal with tweezers is best. Use disinfectant solution on the wound.

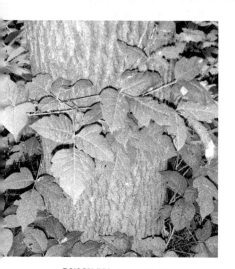

POISON IVY Photographed by Tom Watson

POISON IVY, OAK, AND SUMAC Recognizing and avoiding poison ivy, oak, and sumac is the most effective way to prevent the painful, itchy rashes associated with these plants. Poison ivy occurs as a vine or groundcover, 3 leaflets to a leaf; poison oak occurs as either a vine or shrub, also with 3 leaflets; and poison sumac flourishes in swampland, each leaf having 7–13 leaflets. Urushiol, the oil in the sap of these plants, is responsible for the rash. Within 14 hours of exposure, raised lines and/or blisters will appear on the affected area, accompanied by a terrible itch. Refrain from scratching because bacteria under your fingernails can cause an infection. Wash and dry the affected area thoroughly, applying a calamine lotion to help dry out the rash. If itching or blistering is severe, seek medical attention. If you do come into contact with one of these plants, remember that oil-contaminated clothes, pets, or hiking gear can easily cause an irritating rash on you or someone else, so wash not only any exposed parts of your body but also clothes, gear, and pets if applicable.

Hunting

Separate rules, regulations, and licenses govern the various hunting types and related seasons. Though there are generally no problems, hikers may wish to forgo their trips during the big-game seasons, usually in November and December, when the woods suddenly seem filled with orange and camouflage. Places you may encounter hunters will be the Cherokee and Chattahoochee National Forests and some wildlife management areas through which hiking trails travel, such as Prentice Cooper State Forest.

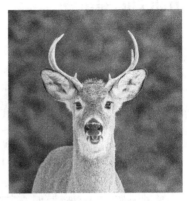

WHITE-TAILED DEER
Photographed by RT Images/Shutterstock

Tips on Enjoying Hiking in Greater Chattanooga

Before you go, read the hike description in this book and visit the website of the intended hiking destination. Call ahead if you have unanswered questions. This will help you get oriented to the forthcoming hike.

Investigate different destinations. The Southern Appalachians may have the highest elevations, but you can literally expand you horizons with a trip to the Cumberland Plateau, or check out a city greenway. Take a chance and make a new adventure instead of trying to recreate the same one over and over. You'll be pleasantly surprised to see so many distinct landscapes in greater Chattanooga.

Take your time along the trails. Pace yourself. Our area is filled with wonders both big and small. Don't rush past a tiny salamander to get to that overlook. Stop and smell the wildflowers. Go ahead and take a seat on a trailside rock. Peer into a stream to find secretive fish. Take pictures. Make memories. Don't miss the trees for the forest.

Timing your hike. We can't always schedule our free time when we want, but try to hike during the week and avoid the traditional holidays if possible. Trails that are packed in the summer are often clear during the colder months. If you are hiking on a busy day, go early in the morning; it'll increase your chances of seeing wildlife. The trails really clear out during rainy times; however, don't hike during a thunderstorm.

Trail Etiquette

Always treat the trail, wildlife, and fellow hikers with respect. Here are some reminders.

* *Plan ahead* in order to be self-sufficient at all times; carry necessary supplies for changes in weather or other conditions. A well-executed trip is a satisfaction to you and to others.

* *Hike on open trails only.*

* *Respect trail and road closures* (ask if not sure), avoid possible trespassing on private land, and obtain all permits and authorization as required. Also, leave gates as you find them or as marked.

* *Be courteous to other hikers,* cyclists, equestrians, and others you encounter on the trails.

* *Never spook animals.* An unannounced approach, a sudden movement, or a loud noise startles most animals. A surprised animal can be dangerous to you, to others, and to itself. Give them plenty of space.

* *Observe the* YIELD *signs* that are displayed around the region's trailheads and backcountry. They advise hikers to yield to horses and bikers to yield to both horses and hikers. A common courtesy on hills is that hikers and bikers yield to any uphill traffic. When encountering mounted riders or horse packers, hikers can courteously step off the trail, on the downhill side if possible. Speak to the riders before they reach you and do not dart behind trees. You are less spooky if the horse can see and hear you. Resist the urge to pet horses unless you are invited to do so.

* *Leave only footprints.* Be sensitive to the ground beneath you. This also means staying on the existing trail and not blazing any new trails.

* *Be sure to pack out what you pack in.* No one likes to see the trash someone else has left behind.

REWARDING HIKES LEAD TO VIEWS LIKE THIS OF THE TENNESSEE RIVER.

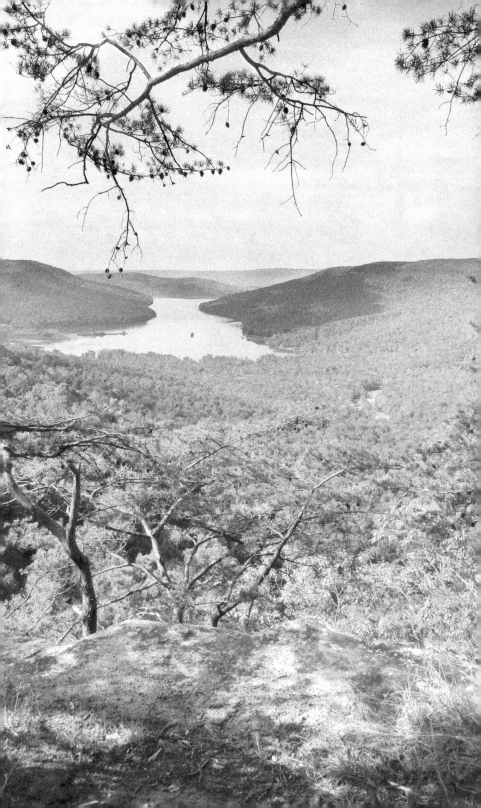

Greater Chattanooga (Hikes 1–13)

Greater Chattanooga

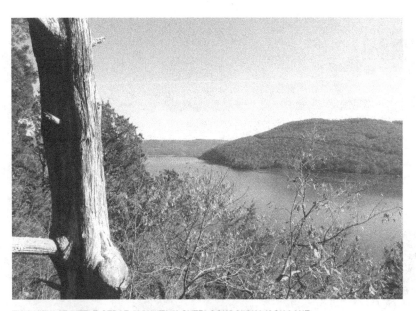

THIS VIEW AT LITTLE CEDAR MOUNTAIN OVERLOOKS NICKAJACK LAKE.
(SEE HIKE 8, PAGE 55)

Harrison Bay State Park:
Bay Point Loop

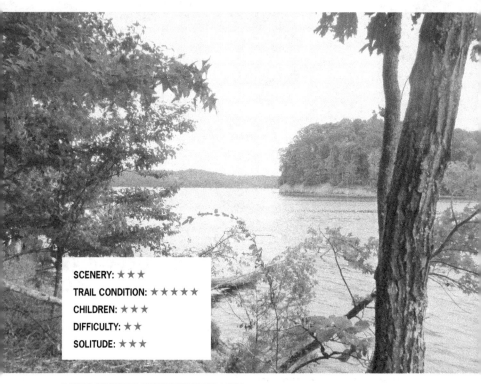

SCENERY: ★ ★ ★
TRAIL CONDITION: ★ ★ ★ ★ ★
CHILDREN: ★ ★ ★
DIFFICULTY: ★ ★
SOLITUDE: ★ ★ ★

A TRAILSIDE VIEW OF CHICKAMAUGA LAKE

GPS TRAILHEAD COORDINATES: N35° 10.095' W85° 07.189'

DISTANCE & CONFIGURATION: 4.2-mile balloon

HIKING TIME: 2 hours

HIGHLIGHTS: Lake views

ELEVATION: 700' at trailhead, 628' at low point

ACCESS: No fees, permits, or passes required

MAPS: *Harrison Bay State Park;* USGS *Snow Hill*

FACILITIES: Restrooms, picnic area, ranger station, restaurant, marina, campground

WHEELCHAIR ACCESS: None

CONTACTS: Harrison Bay State Park, 423-344-6214, tnstateparks.com

Overview

This easy, nearly level loop trail at Harrison Bay State Park winds along the shores of Chickamauga Lake amid a series of peninsulas jutting into the huge Tennessee Valley Authority (TVA) impoundment. While hiking, you will stay along the shore for most of the route, soaking in scenic lake vistas one after another. While here, consider enjoying the other amenities of this preserve, including paddling, boating, picnicking, and camping.

Route Details

Harrison Bay State Park was Tennessee's first state park, opened in 1937 originally as a TVA recreation area set on the shores of Chickamauga Lake, a dammed portion of the Tennessee River. The name *Harrison Bay* came from the former community of Harrison, which was covered by the lake when it was filled in the 1930s. Where once was Harrison is now Harrison Bay. Parts of the community are still visible, however, in the form of islands rising above the impoundment, and miles of shoreline were created, almost 40 miles in the park alone!

The natural question is this: How do you get 40 miles of shoreline in a 1,200-acre park? Answer: The park is composed of multiple peninsulas jutting into the lake, one after another, and is literally almost all shoreline. You will travel a series of these peninsulas on this hike. These ridges are low, making the hike an easy proposition, especially considering the fine state of the trails, so you don't have to watch every footfall and can enjoy looking at the water, islands, and miles of tan sand beaches.

Although the trail is open to bicycles, you won't find many two-wheelers on the path—the trail is too easy for hardcore mountain bikers, leaving only the occasional bicycling camper to roll through the Bay Point Loop. For hikers, this well-marked and maintained path is excellent for daily exercise, and you can shorten it if desired. Not only will you experience continual views between the trailside trees, but you will also travel to cleared views replete with contemplation benches.

The trailhead signboard displays interpretive information about the natural components of the forest. Pick up the Bay Point Loop, entering woods of cedar, pine, sycamore, and sweetgum. The path quickly splits. Head right,

Harrison Bay State Park: Bay Point Loop

making a counterclockwise loop. The woods are level enough here to have vernal pools that form during winter and last into spring before drying out, only to repeat the cycle as the seasons come and go. Curve near a cove of Chickamauga

Lake, viewing the park marina. Ahead you will reach the first cleared view, where you'll also find a shaded bench. Look west into the bay of the marina, as well as at park islands and peninsulas. In season, watercraft from kayaks to johnboats to sailboats, pontoon boats, and yachts will be plying the waters. If you are into kayaking or canoeing, the shore and islands of this state park are fine to explore. Continuing on the path, you will pass unofficial spur trails leading to other overlooks as well as beaches. As the lake recedes after reaching its spring high water, sandier shoreline will be exposed.

At 0.4 mile, pass a shortcut leading left to a boardwalk. By 0.9 mile, you will have circled the first peninsula of the trail. The next peninsula has more vertical variation—a few hills. Continue to enjoy view after view circling this second peninsula. At 1.5 miles, you are at the southern tip of the second peninsula, as pines spill their needles onto the trailbed. At 1.8 miles, you reach another bench and overlook. From there, head north along a long, slim cove. Stay with the cove, reaching the other end of the boardwalk that you passed earlier at 2.2 miles, and head over one of the aforementioned vernal pools, seasonal wetlands that will be high and dry in summer and fall. Curve around to the north end of the cove and reach the third and final peninsula. This third peninsula is the longest and the largest. At 3.1 miles you'll arrive at the most southerly point of this peninsula and a view. Gaze out on Patten Island, TN 58, and the balance of Harrison Bay. Continue curving along the shore while a piney hill rises on the center of this peninsula. By 3.9 miles you have left the lake and are wandering north in thick woods. At 4.1 miles you complete the loop portion of the hike. A backtrack leads to the trailhead and hike's end.

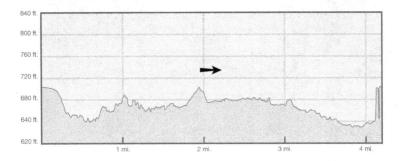

Nearby Attractions

Harrison Bay State Park has a boat ramp; marina; boat, canoe, and kayak rentals; a camp store; a restaurant; a swimming pool; birding; fishing; picnicking; camping; and even golf.

Directions

From Exit 11 on I-75 near Ooltewah, Tennessee, take US 11/US 64 west 0.3 mile to turn left onto Hunter Road, then follow Hunter Road 6.1 miles to reach TN 58. From there, turn right and join TN 58 for 1.5 miles to turn left onto Harrison Bay Road. Follow Harrison Bay Road 1.5 miles to enter the state park. From there, follow the signs to the marina/boat ramp to the end of the road near the park office. From the ramp area, curve east into a large parking lot. The signed Bay Point Loop Trailhead is at the east end of the large parking lot.

THIS INVITING TRACK LEADS YOU PAST WATERY VISTAS APLENTY.

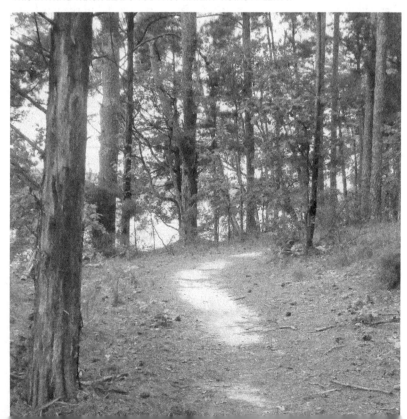

2

Greenway Farms Park

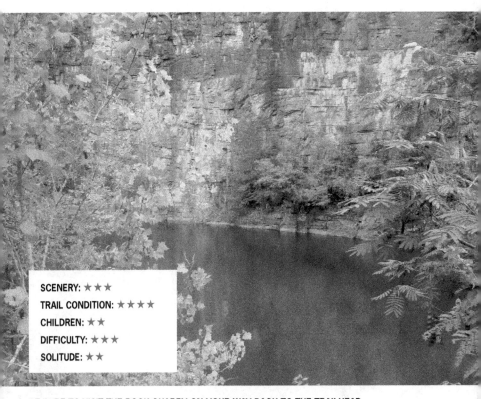

SCENERY: ★ ★ ★
TRAIL CONDITION: ★ ★ ★ ★
CHILDREN: ★ ★
DIFFICULTY: ★ ★ ★
SOLITUDE: ★ ★

BE SURE TO VISIT THE ROCK QUARRY ON YOUR WAY BACK TO THE TRAILHEAD.

GPS TRAILHEAD COORDINATES: N35° 07.724' W85° 12.899'

DISTANCE & CONFIGURATION: 6.2-mile triple balloon

HIKING TIME: 3.4 hours

HIGHLIGHTS: TVA Small Wild Area, views, rock quarry

ELEVATION: 680' at trailhead, 1,001' at high point

ACCESS: No fees, permits, or passes required

MAPS: *Greenway Farms—North Chickamauga Creek Conservancy, TVA Big Ridge Trail;* USGS *Daisy, East Chattanooga*

FACILITIES: Restrooms, dog park, paddler accesses, rental facilities

WHEELCHAIR ACCESS: Along greenway

CONTACTS: Greenway Farms Park, 423-643-6311, chattanooga.gov

Greenway Farms Park

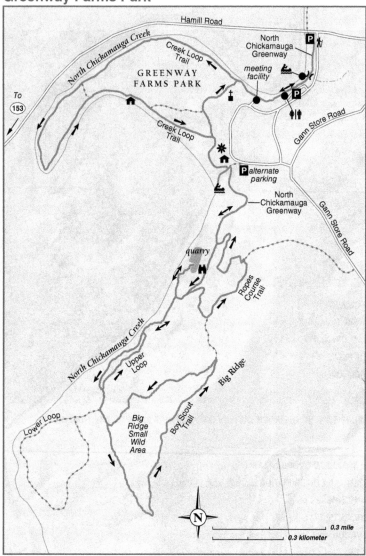

Overview

This hike combines a Chattanooga city park and a Tennessee Valley Authority (TVA) wild tract to form a fun and interesting trek. Start by walking along North Chickamauga Creek at Greenway Farms Park; enjoy the stream scenes.

Leave the water to climb Big Ridge, where surprising panoramas await. Next, enter TVA's Big Ridge Small Wild Area, climbing to the hike's high point in big woods. Stop by a small lake and rock quarry on your return trip to the trailhead.

Route Details

This hike combines not only two parks in one adventure but also lots of different types of trails. The downside may be the myriad trail intersections, but if you get lost for a minute, just ask for help from your fellow hikers you are sure to see at this popular destination. Take a photo of the map in this guide before you set out. Not only will you take different trails, from singletrack footpaths to paved greenways, but you will also savor streams, a lake, distant views, towering trees, and even an old cemetery. After coming here a few times, you may want to create your own hike within the trail network. However, the suggested hike heads to all the highlights.

The adventure first joins gravel North Chickamauga Greenway, heading south into Greenway Farms Park. You bridge a little tributary, then pass one of the kayak/canoe accesses on North Chickamauga Creek. Walk behind a park restroom before reaching an intersection at 0.3 mile. Here, leave right onto the natural-surface Creek Loop Trail. The flat track traces the bends of North Chickamauga Creek. This flat was prime farmland before the land became a park in 1990. Formerly, crops were grown, cattle were run, and it was once even a dairy farm before being bought by a dentist and then sold to the city. Now forest has reclaimed the fields, while other areas are being cultivated in native grasses and wildflowers.

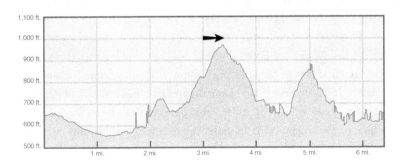

At 0.8 mile, a spur heads left, shortcutting the Creek Loop Trail. You keep straight, tunneling under trees and passing the other end of the shortcut at 1.3 miles. Ahead, you will view an old cabin by the creek before returning to the North Chickamauga Greenway at 1.7 miles. Turn right onto the now-paved trail, coming near developed gardens and another cabin. At a four-way intersection, first head right at the kayak/canoe access to see the creek one more time, then continue on the greenway. Ahead you will climb Big Ridge. At 2.2 miles, the Ropes Course Trail leaves left, but you stay straight, climbing to discover a view above a water-filled quarry, created when limestone was obtained for the construction of nearby Chickamauga Dam on the Tennessee River back in the 1930s. From the overlook, Walden Ridge forms the western horizon. Ahead, descend past the other end of the Ropes Course Trail and a spur that heads right to the quarry, both of which you will hike upon your return. At 2.5 miles the North Chickamauga Greenway divides; stay with the Lower Loop.

At 2.7 miles, the trail merges, and you enter TVA's 200-acre Big Ridge Small Wild Area. One of 28 special parcels of TVA property, Big Ridge was originally part of the land purchase for the quarry. But the forest here caught TVA's attention, and the tulip trees, shagbark hickory, and oaks were preserved as a place for wildlife and also trails for us.

Pick up the singletrack, natural-surface Boy Scout Trail, climbing from the paved greenway. Stay right, as the Boy Scout Trail divides to fashion a loop. Crest out on Big Ridge, scanning for old-growth trees. At 3.5 miles stay left as a connector trail leaves right for the Ropes Course Trail. Complete the Boy Scout Loop at 3.9 miles, then backtrack the North Chickamauga Greenway, staying right with the Upper Loop. Ahead, the greenway comes together, and you are backtracking again. At 4.6 miles, head left on a spur trail to explore the rock quarry. You may see anglers down here in the still tarn backed by sheer stone walls. Backtrack to the North Chickamauga Greenway, and then head right with the natural-surface Ropes Course Trail (just a hiking trail these days) at 4.8 miles. Wind into woods, meeting the spur to the Boy Scout Trail and then a connector to Gann Store Road before dropping to intersect the North Chickamauga Greenway again at 5.2 miles. From here you descend off Big Ridge, backtracking on the greenway. At 5.5 miles you return to the four-way intersection where you were earlier, near the gardens and cabin. Keep straight, picking up a new segment of greenway. Walk among open grasses to pass a cemetery on a hill to your right, where the graves of farm families lie. You'll reach the Creek Loop ahead. Make a final backtrack, returning to the trailhead at 6.2 miles, having explored the highlights and highpoints of Greenway Farms Park and Big Ridge Small Wild Area.

Nearby Attractions

In addition to trails, this preserve has a dog park and paddler accesses for plying North Chickamauga Creek, as well as picnic areas and rental facilities for groups.

Directions

From Exit 4 on I-75 northeast of Chattanooga, take TN 153 north 7.8 miles, crossing the Tennessee River. Turn right onto Hamill Road and follow it 1.6 miles. Turn right into Greenway Farms Park, just after bridging North Chicka-mauga Creek, then continue a short distance to turn right into the first parking area in the park. Here, you join the North Chickamauga Greenway.

3

Riverwalk at Chickamauga Dam

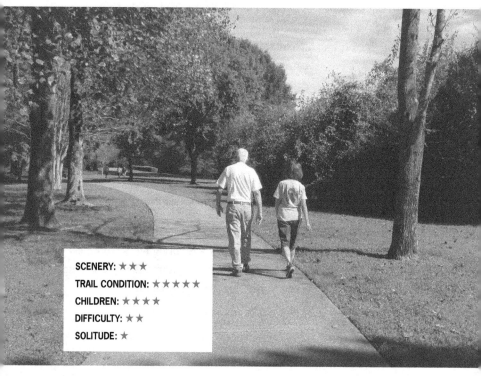

SCENERY: ★ ★ ★
TRAIL CONDITION: ★ ★ ★ ★ ★
CHILDREN: ★ ★ ★ ★
DIFFICULTY: ★ ★
SOLITUDE: ★

THE RIVERWALK IS IDEAL AS A SCENIC REGULAR WALKING DESTINATION.

GPS TRAILHEAD COORDINATES: N35° 06.133' W85° 13.827'

DISTANCE & CONFIGURATION: 3-mile out-and-back

HIKING TIME: 1.8 hours

HIGHLIGHTS: Tennessee River views, trailside art, fishing, picnicking

ELEVATION: 640' at trailhead, 660' at high point

ACCESS: No fees, permits, or passes required

MAPS: *Tennessee Riverpark;* USGS *East Chattanooga, Chattanooga*

FACILITIES: Restroom, benches near trailhead

WHEELCHAIR ACCESS: Yes

CONTACTS: Tennessee Riverpark, 423-493-9239, parks.hamiltontn.gov

Overview

Enjoy a slice of Chattanooga's nationally renowned greenway—Riverwalk. Start on its eastern end, just below Chickamauga Dam, and walk amid landscaped grounds overlooking the mighty Tennessee River. Along the way, pass through a large green space enhanced with outdoor art. Make a little loop through Fishing Park, with its numerous angling piers extending into the water, before returning to Chickamauga Dam.

Route Details

Chattanooga's Riverwalk is a nationally acclaimed model not only as an exercise and hiking destination but also as a way to enhance river frontage and gather the community. Its actual name is Tennessee Riverpark, but the term *Riverwalk* has superseded the original in common nomenclature. In the early 1980s, the idea was born to build a linear preserve along the Tennessee River, extending from Chickamauga Dam to Lookout Mountain. The original plan was unveiled in 1985. Citizens and government personnel all realized the creation of the Riverwalk would come in stages, just as the building of the Appalachian Trail was a section-by-section endeavor.

And so goes Riverwalk. This particular section travels from Chickamauga Dam to Fishing Park, the first section of path to be built. It opened in 1989. The trail currently extends to downtown Chattanooga and Lookout Mountain. It has been an incredible success, so much so that the newest sections are the widest segments of trail yet, built to accommodate a high volume of hikers, joggers, bicyclists, and other outdoors enthusiasts.

As magnificent as the Riverwalk is, it is but one greenway in an ever-expanding system of linear trails coursing through greater Chattanooga. The North Chickamauga Creek Greenway and the South Chickamauga Creek Greenway come to mind. Stay tuned for more expansion while enjoying the current open segments, including this one.

After parking as close to Chickamauga Dam as possible, begin following the Tennessee River on a series of the sidewalks bordered with picnic tables, benches, and more. Absorb the interpretive and historical information about the Tennessee River, the Chickamauga Dam, and the park through which you

Riverwalk at Chickamauga Dam

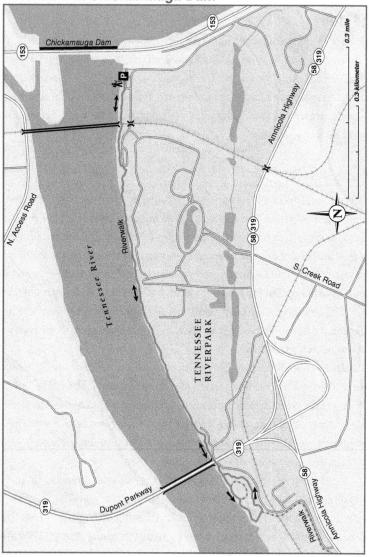

walk. Shortly pass under a railroad bridge, then reach a fishing pier and boat ramp after a quarter mile. This first segment can be busy with all sorts of park enthusiasts rather than just trail users. Beyond here, the path passes a shaded pavilion, leaving the dam tailwater area, and becomes more of a pure trail-centered greenway.

Here, you continue west, traveling the asphalt track with the river to your right and Chattanooga State Community College to your left. Some trail sections are shaded, and some are not. Note the mileages of the Tennessee River embedded into the trail itself. These measurements are given in quarter-mile increments. Occasional shade shelters and contemplation benches are placed along the path. River views are nearly continuous. Surprisingly, the trail does have a little vertical variation, though the ups and downs are slight.

At 0.8 mile, the Riverwalk bridges a stream and opens onto an expansive green space, dotted with trees and trailside art. These sculptures and designs add a creative element to the park and greenway. See, the Riverwalk isn't simply a nature trail; rather, it is an agglomeration of green space, pathway, and public square. Art enhances the landscape much as other elements of any park. Befitting the scene, many of the art pieces have a water or river theme.

The open green space closes as you pass under DuPont Parkway. However, this is where you enter aptly named Fishing Park. Notice the multiple piers extending into the water to enhance the angling experience. It's fun to just sit awhile and watch the anglers tussle with the finned critters. Beyond the piers, Fishing Park has a central amphitheater along with a network of short interconnected paths and picnic areas that create a gathering space for park users, not necessarily only Riverwalk hikers. The park even has an on-site concessionaire selling food in season. Even though the trails at Fishing Park seem a maze, you can make a loop on your return trip. The Riverwalk continues westerly from Fishing Park but turns away from the river near the boat ramp, at 1.5 miles.

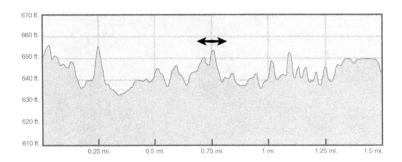

The next greenway section stretches 1 mile to a place called Riverpoint, where South Chickamauga Creek flows into the Tennessee River. From there, it's about 5 miles to the downtown area. Eventually, the South Chickamauga Creek Greenway will connect to Riverwalk near Riverpoint. Enjoy wandering through Fishing Park before backtracking to the Chickamauga Dam Trailhead.

Nearby Attractions

Chickamauga Lake is a water lover's paradise, with swimming, fishing, boating, and other aquatic recreation.

Directions

From Exit 4 on I-75, northeast of downtown Chattanooga, take TN 153 north 5.3 miles to TN 319, Amnicola Highway. Exit north on TN 319 and follow it 6 miles to the right turn to the Riverpark–Chickamauga Dam segment. Follow the entrance road 0.3 mile, then veer left onto another road with a sign that reads RIVERPARK RECREATION. Follow this road to park at the dam tailwater area.

4 South Chickamauga Battlefield Loop

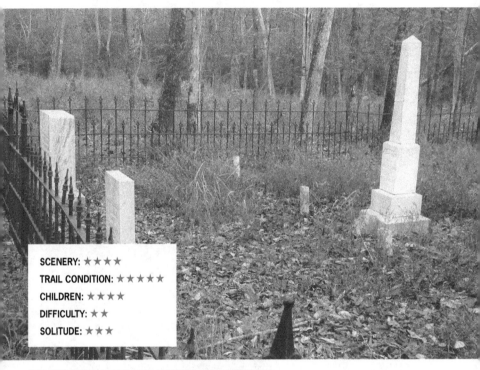

SCENERY: ★ ★ ★ ★
TRAIL CONDITION: ★ ★ ★ ★ ★
CHILDREN: ★ ★ ★ ★
DIFFICULTY: ★ ★
SOLITUDE: ★ ★ ★

THIS HIKE TAKES YOU BY THE HISTORIC HUNT CEMETERY.

GPS TRAILHEAD COORDINATES: N34° 56.364' W85° 15.582'
DISTANCE & CONFIGURATION: 4.1-mile loop
HIKING TIME: 2.5 hours
HIGHLIGHTS: Civil War battlefield, West Chickamauga Creek, rare cedar glades
ELEVATION: 750' at trailhead, 700' at low point
ACCESS: No fees, permits, or passes required
MAPS: *Chickamauga Battlefield Trails; USGS Fort Oglethorpe, East Ridge*
FACILITIES: None
WHEELCHAIR ACCESS: None
CONTACTS: Chickamauga & Chattanooga National Military Park, 706-866-9241, nps.gov/chch

South Chickamauga Battlefield Loop

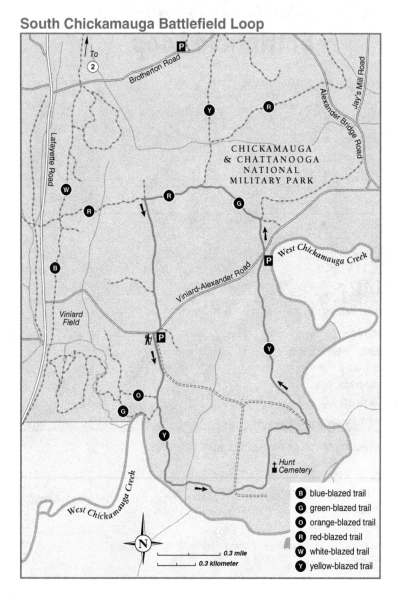

CHICKAMAUGA
& CHATTANOOGA
NATIONAL
MILITARY PARK

West Chickamauga Creek

Viniard-Alexander Road

Lafayette Road

Brotherton Road

Alexander Bridge Road

Jay's Mill Road

Viniard
Field

West Chickamauga Creek

Hunt
Cemetery

To 2

N

0.3 mile
0.3 kilometer

B blue-blazed trail
G green-blazed trail
O orange-blazed trail
R red-blazed trail
W white-blazed trail
Y yellow-blazed trail

Overview

This hike explores the southeastern, wild, and natural side of Chickamauga Battlefield, all within a gigantic bend of West Chickamauga Creek. First, wander through rich woods to come along the attractive stream. The hike then bisects forest and meadow, passing Hunt Cemetery. Hike along drainages of West Chickamauga Creek, then rise to limestone uplands where open cedar glades form a unique environment with rare flora. Finally, pass some monuments and Civil War history before closing the loop.

Route Details

The most southeasterly part of Chickamauga Battlefield, located just south of Fort Oglethorpe, Georgia, seems more like a protected nature park than a place where the Union and Confederacy clashed for control of Chattanooga, a strategic city for transportation and the gateway to the lower South. Even during that eventful September in 1863, when thousands of men risked their lives for their respective causes, this area was a backwater. In fact, when the boundaries of the battlefield were laid out, West Chickamauga Creek made for a convenient line. This big bend added to the acreage, thus protecting some scenic and biologically important woodlands through which we can hike.

Speaking of boundaries, did you know that Chickamauga & Chattanooga National Military Park was the first US national park established to protect a Civil War site? Back in 1888, after the establishment of Yellowstone National Park, people began to see the national park model as a way to preserve significant historical sites, as well as superlatively beautiful natural locations. Just a quarter century after the battle, a pair of generals toured the battlefields and recommended preservation at both Lookout Mountain and Chickamauga. Congressional approval came in 1890, and the park was dedicated on September 18, 1895, 32 years to the day after the clash.

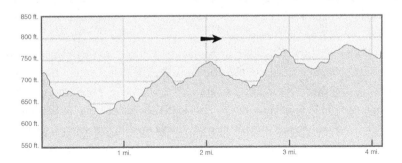

Men who had participated in the campaign helped lay out the memorials and provided strategic information. They are responsible for what we see today not only from a military perspective; preserving large battlefields meant setting aside acreage, which led to the creation of a natural preserve.

The battlefield trails are unnamed but color coded. Red, blue, and white paths are open to horses and hiking, whereas the yellow, green, and orange paths are hiker only. Despite all the twists and turns, the trails are well marked, and the color maps available at the visitor center are very helpful.

Begin your hike by following the roadbed behind a pole gate heading south. Follow the old route through woods before reaching a yellow-blazed trail at 0.2 mile. Turn right here, following a narrower hiker-only track. Hickory, pine, redbud, and cedar, as well as some oaks, rise above the limestone-heavy soil. At 0.3 mile an orange-blazed trail leaves right. Stay with the yellow-blazed trail under bigger trees. This is a quiet part of the park. At 0.7 mile you'll come alongside West Chickamauga Creek. A short spur trail leads to the waterway. Gain a rewarding look at this large creek, which flows quietly at this point. Sycamore, paw paw, and hackberry fill the bottomland. Curve easterly, keeping in the bottoms. This is a good spring wildflower area.

Open onto a field at 1 mile. Stay with the right-hand side of the clearing. Just ahead, briefly pick up a roadbed and look for the yellow-blazed hiker trail, continuing easterly. At 1.3 miles open onto another field. Turn left here, northbound. Come to the wrought iron–encircled Hunt Cemetery at 1.4 miles. Prebattle residents are interred here.

Hickories, pines, and cedars continue to dominate the low hills. At 1.8 miles cross a closed park road and keep north, still with the hiker-only, yellow-blazed trail. The path descends along a tributary of West Chickamauga Creek. Pass through bottoms of beard cane, then cross Viniard-Alexander Road at 2.7 miles. Limestone slabs open in the woodlands.

You soon enter full-blown limestone cedar glades. At first glance, these rare plant communities seem like crumbly old parking lots with a few weeds growing atop them, but in fact they are very rare in Georgia and from a global perspective can be found only in a few places in the southeastern United States, with Middle Tennessee being the heart of their range. In late summer you will see the rare Tennessee coneflower and Tennessee gladecress, among many other plants unique to the community.

These cedar glades are easily the most biologically significant plant communities within the battlefield. Fast-draining, thin soils open to the sun leave these glades to all but a few specialized plants. Even the cedar trees are stunted! At 2.8 miles a large cedar glade appears on your left. Just ahead look left and join a green-blazed trail meandering northwesterly through occasional small glades. At 3.2 miles stay left, joining a red-blazed path, heading west in mature deep woods. Come to a four-way junction at 3.5 miles. Turn left here, back on a yellow-blazed path. Pass more limestone pockets and some battlefield monuments. The level path leads you to Viniard-Alexander Road and the end of your loop. The parking area is within sight to the right.

Nearby Attractions

The 5,300-acre Chickamauga Battlefield offers more miles of hiking and equestrian trails, historical buildings, and a 7-mile auto tour with additional roads for seeing the battlefield. The visitor center has numerous exhibits, a video describing the battlefield, a detailed battlefield map, historical artifacts, and military items, including a special collection of shoulder arms.

Directions

From Exit 350 on I-75 in Georgia, southeast of downtown Chattanooga, take GA 2/Battlefield Parkway west 6.4 miles to Fort Oglethorpe, Georgia, and Lafayette Road. Turn left on Lafayette Road and follow it 1 mile to reach the visitor center on your right. (You may want to stop in and obtain a trail map.) Continue past the visitor center 2.5 more miles, then turn left on Viniard-Alexander Road. Follow Viniard-Alexander Road 0.7 mile to a parking area on your right.

North Chickamauga Battlefield Loop

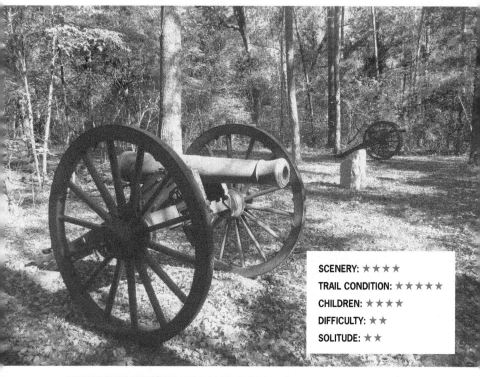

SCENERY: ★ ★ ★ ★
TRAIL CONDITION: ★ ★ ★ ★ ★
CHILDREN: ★ ★ ★ ★
DIFFICULTY: ★ ★
SOLITUDE: ★ ★

CANNON EMPLACEMENTS MARK POSITIONS OF UNION AND CONFEDERATE FORCES.

GPS TRAILHEAD COORDINATES: N34° 56.364' W85° 15.582'

DISTANCE & CONFIGURATION: 4.8-mile double loop

HIKING TIME: 3 hours

HIGHLIGHTS: Civil War battlefield, monuments, interpretive signage

ELEVATION: 740' at trailhead, 790' at high point

ACCESS: No fees, permits, or passes required

MAPS: *Chickamauga Battlefield Trails;* USGS *Fort Oglethorpe, East Ridge*

FACILITIES: Visitor center, restroom, fountain

WHEELCHAIR ACCESS: None

CONTACTS: Chickamauga & Chattanooga National Military Park, 706-866-9241, nps.gov/chch

Overview

This mostly level hike starts at Chickamauga Battlefield visitor center, then explores the hills, creeks, forests, and, of course, the monuments and historical features of this Civil War site. Cross Black Creek, then turn east near Reed's Bridge Road. The trail then passes battlefield lines and monuments before coming to the site of Jay's Mill. Wander through woods to reach Brotherton Road, with interpretive information aplenty. The hike then makes its way through more mixed fields and woods, and human and natural history, before returning to the visitor center. The hike is free of climbs, and the expansive trail network allows you to shorten or lengthen the walk.

Route Details

During the Civil War both the Union and the Confederacy prized the city of Chattanooga. Strategically located along the Tennessee River and a railroad crossroad, the city was key to the Confederates in defending the lower South and to the Federals in continuing their plan to split the South in two. Chickamauga Battlefield, located just south of Fort Oglethorpe, Georgia, was the location of the last major Confederate victory. Later that fall, in Chattanooga, the Union ultimately cracked the Confederate defenses, enabling Sherman's infamous March to the Sea.

During your hike you will see monuments erected to various troops on both sides. You will also see plaques helping to explain the complex movements during the September 1863 clash. However, a trip to the visitor center at the trailhead will give you a much more comprehensive understanding of the battle than you'll get from walking through one particular area of the national military park. So consider it a mixture of enjoying nature as well as history.

The battlefield trails are unnamed but color coded. Red, blue, and white paths are open to horses and hiking, whereas the yellow, green, and orange paths are hiker only. Despite all the twists and turns, the trails are well marked, and the color maps available at the visitor center are very helpful. The hike leaves south from the visitor center parking lot, passing through a grassy field. You'll soon reach an intersection just before a wooden footbridge. Turn left on a red-blazed trail to pass under Lafayette Road at the culvert where Black Creek flows

North Chickamauga Battlefield Loop

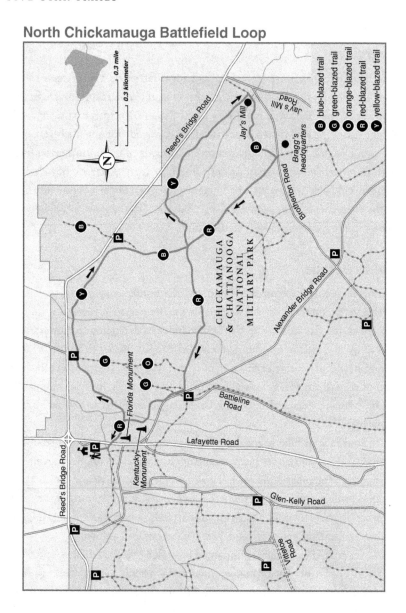

under the road. If the water is high, just cross on the road. At 0.2 mile look left for a yellow-blazed trail. Take this hiker-only path to enter flatwoods of hickory, pine, cedar, and oak. Despite the fact that you are in deep woods, civilization hums in the background. At 0.6 mile reach a four-way intersection. Here, you can see a parking area to your left at Reed's Bridge Road. Keep straight on the yellow-blazed trail, roughly paralleling the curves of Reed's Bridge Road. Dip to span another tributary of Black Creek at 0.9 mile. At 1.4 miles stay straight on a blue-blazed trail.

Pass your first battlefield monuments before reaching a four-way intersection at 1.6 miles. Turn left here, joining another yellow-blazed, hiker-only trail. You will return to this intersection later. The rocky path continues paralleling Reed's Bridge Road, heading downhill toward the site of Jay's Mill, on West Chickamauga Creek in tall pines. At 2.5 miles make an abrupt right just before reaching Jay's Mill Road. Join a blue-blazed path heading right. Step over a limestone-bedded streamlet and travel sinkhole-pocked land. Cedars, redbuds, and hickories thrive in this limestone soil. At 2.9 miles emerge very near Brotherton Road, not far from Confederate General Braxton Bragg's headquarters. However, this loop does not cross Brotherton Road (but that shouldn't stop you should you wish to detour to the site of Bragg's headquarters). Instead, turn right on a red-blazed trail, heading northwest. Spur trails lead from this path, exploring other monuments and interpretive battlefield information. These spurs can add to your mileage and learning experience.

At 3.5 miles return to the four-way intersection where you were earlier. Stay left, still with the red-blazed trail. At 4 miles step over the headwaters of Black Creek. Keep west in an area with many monuments. Allow ample time for your hike, as you will be attracted to all of this interpretive information. At 4.2 miles you will reach Alexander Bridge Road. Stay with the red-blazed trail as it turns north, staying very close to Alexander Bridge Road. Open onto a field at 4.5 miles. The Florida Monument and visitor center are visible in the distance.

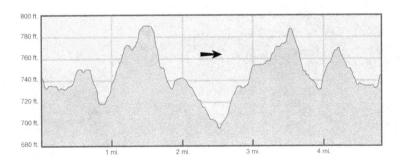

The path stays along the field's edge, effectively half-circling the Florida Monument. The last 0.2 mile of the hike is a backtrack. Finish your trek at 4.8 miles.

Nearby Attractions

The 5,300-acre Chickamauga Battlefield offers more miles of hiking and equestrian trails, historical buildings, and a 7-mile auto tour with additional roads for seeing the battlefield. The visitor center has numerous exhibits, a video describing the battlefield, a detailed battlefield map, historical artifacts, and military items, including a special collection of shoulder arms.

Directions

From Exit 350 on I-75 in Georgia, southeast of downtown Chattanooga, take GA 2/Battlefield Parkway west 6.4 miles to Fort Oglethorpe, Georgia, and Lafayette Road. Turn left on Lafayette Road and follow it 1 mile to reach the visitor center on your right. The large visitor parking area is just south of the visitor center. The hike starts here (if you pass the Florida Monument on your left you have gone just a little too far).

FIELDS ARE KEPT AS THEY WERE IN 1863, WITH INFORMATIVE MONUMENTS ADDED.

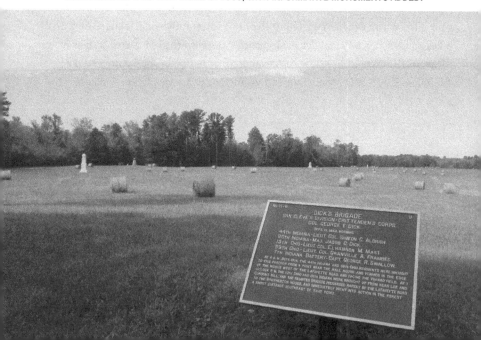

6 Cravens House Loop

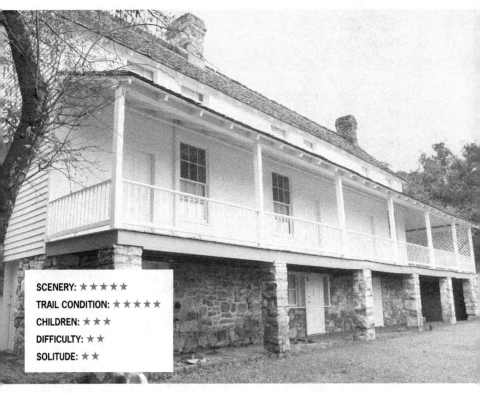

SCENERY: ★ ★ ★ ★ ★
TRAIL CONDITION: ★ ★ ★ ★ ★
CHILDREN: ★ ★ ★
DIFFICULTY: ★ ★
SOLITUDE: ★ ★

THE CRAVENS HOUSE IS A HIGHLIGHT OF THIS HIKE.

GPS TRAILHEAD COORDINATES: N35° 00.590' W85° 20.626'

DISTANCE & CONFIGURATION: 2.6-mile balloon

HIKING TIME: 1.5 hours

HIGHLIGHTS: Civil War history, expansive vistas, the Cravens House

ELEVATION: 2,110' at trailhead, 1,570' at low point

ACCESS: Entrance fee required

MAPS: *Lookout Mountain Trail Map;* USGS *Chattanooga*

FACILITIES: Visitor center, restrooms, picnic area at trailhead

WHEELCHAIR ACCESS: On upper part of Point Park

CONTACTS: Chickamauga & Chattanooga National Military Park, 706-866-9241, nps.gov/chch

Cravens House Loop

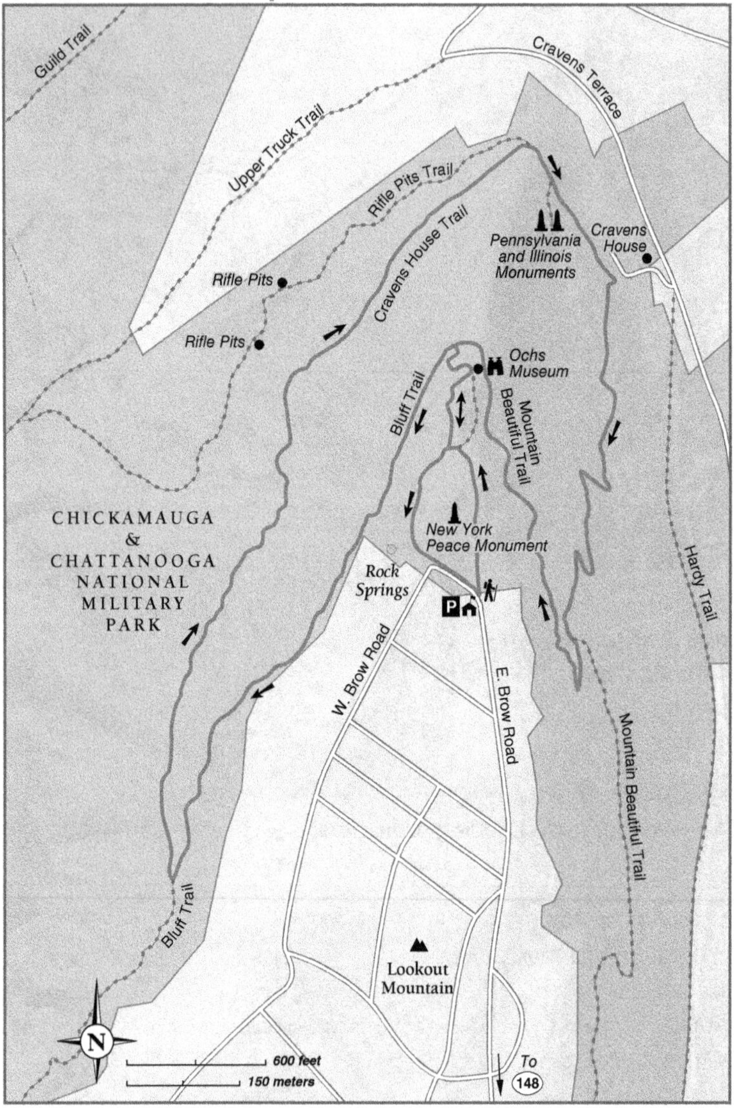

Guild Trail

Cravens Terrace

Upper Truck Trail

Rifle Pits Trail

Cravens House Trail

Pennsylvania and Illinois Monuments

Cravens House

Rifle Pits

Rifle Pits

Ochs Museum

Bluff Trail

Mountain Beautiful Trail

CHICKAMAUGA
&
CHATTANOOGA
NATIONAL
MILITARY
PARK

New York Peace Monument

Rock Springs

Hardy Trail

W. Brow Road

E. Brow Road

Mountain Beautiful Trail

Bluff Trail

Lookout Mountain

N

600 feet
150 meters

To
148

Overview

This hike starts at view-laden Point Park on Lookout Mountain. Wander through the monuments and cannon formations near inspiring views. Drop to Ochs Museum and incredible vistas of Chattanooga. A steady downgrade takes you to the Cravens House, an important Civil War site, with its own panoramas. From there, take a narrow foot access up to the Mountain Beautiful Trail, returning to Point Park. The hike's short distance makes the 500-foot elevation change more tolerable to novice walkers.

Route Details

Civil War history can be found all over greater Chattanooga. And it is atop Lookout Mountain that this history mingles with the natural beauty of the Scenic City. The preservation of important Civil War sites as part of the greater Chattanooga and Chickamauga National Battlefield has not only saved these historic sites, but also the hiking trails located on them add up to miles and miles of possibilities for history buffs, hikers, bicyclists, and equestrians, all within easy access for Chattanooga's residents.

This hike combines exploration of Civil War history with the beauty of Lookout Mountain. After making your way to Point Park, take a minute to explore the visitor center and pay your entrance fee. Enter the fortresslike gate of Point Park and take the stone slab path downhill. Incredible views open of the flatlands and hills beyond Lookout Mountain. Cannon ramparts lure you to their overlooks. At the bottom of the green space, take the steps leading down toward Ochs Museum. Stone steps lead to the small museum, located on a rock outcrop with perhaps the finest views anywhere in the region. Below, the Tennessee River makes its Moccasin Bend. Signal Mountain and the Cumberland Plateau rise to the left. Chattanooga stretches across the riverside flats and beyond.

Descend from Ochs Museum on metal stairs past a sheer cliff, at the base of which stands a monument laid into the bluff. This is also the site of the

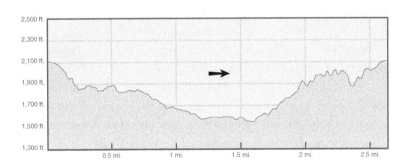

short-lived Point Hotel, which took advantage of the views here. Begin the loop portion of the hike by heading left on the Bluff Trail, toward Sunset Rock. The Mountain Beautiful Trail, your return route, heads right. The Bluff Trail turns southerly beneath incredible rock bluffs and rock houses (natural rock shelters) while sporting winter views of Lookout Valley below.

At 0.4 mile pass developed Rock Springs, located in a cliff alcove on your left. Feast on more big boulders and other geological wonders. At 0.8 mile intersect the Cravens House Trail. Turn acutely right here, northbound, tracing a fairly wide track more downhill than not. Great oak forests rise among the slopes, as do boulders and occasional outcrops.

Curve north past the point of Lookout Mountain, reaching a trail junction at 1.5 miles. Here, the Rifle Pits Trail leads left, but our hike stays right, aiming for the Cravens House. Walk just a short distance, then reach another trail junction. Here a spur leads up to the Illinois and Pennsylvania Monuments. Continue forward to reach the Cravens House at 1.6 miles. The home sits on a brow looking north over Chattanooga. A massive monument stands to the left.

Once you have been here, the house and monument are easily recognizable any time you peer up at Lookout Mountain from the city of Chattanooga. This house headquartered Civil War generals on both sides. It played a significant role in the 1863 Battle Above the Clouds but only suffered minor damage. Later, Union troops destroyed the house. When Robert Cravens returned, he rebuilt his home on the foundations where it stood, and that is the house you see today. The home is accessible by automobile.

To loop back to Point Park, take the steep spur trail leading from the left-hand corner of the homesite as you have your back to the Cravens House. There may be a sign indicating TO MOUNTAIN BEAUTIFUL TRAIL. The narrow path heads uphill. Stay left when it splits at 1.8 miles (a faint, unmaintained trail leads right). Continue switchbacking uphill. A wooden staircase keeps the uptick going. At 2 miles intersect the Mountain Beautiful Trail. Turn right and head northeast along a cliffline. Begin circling below Point Park. At 2.4 miles you have completed the loop portion of the hike. From here, climb the metal stairs to Ochs Museum, grab one more view, then take the stone steps to Point Park. Circle up through Point Park, taking a different route to soak in more views and history, emerging at the stone entrance to the park at 2.6 miles.

Nearby Attractions

The greater Lookout Mountain part of the national battlefield has miles of trails on public lands extending on the east and west sides of the mountain, even into Georgia.

Directions

From Exit 175 on I-24 west of downtown Chattanooga, take Browns Ferry Road south 0.4 mile to a traffic light and Cummings Highway/US 41/64/11/72. Turn left on Cummings Highway and follow it 0.8 mile to turn right on Alford Hill Drive. Follow Alford Hill Drive to soon reach Old Wauhatchie Pike/TN 318. Turn left on Old Wauhatchie Pike and follow it 1.4 miles to reach Scenic Highway/ TN 148. Turn right on Scenic Highway and follow it 2.3 miles, then veer sharply right on East Brow Road (look for signs to Point Park). Follow East Brow Road 1.1 miles to reach Point Park. Parking is on your left just after curving left past the stone Point Park entrance.

THE CASTLELIKE ENTRANCE OF POINT PARK REPRESENTS THE INSIGNIA OF THE U.S. ARMY CORPS OF ENGINEERS.

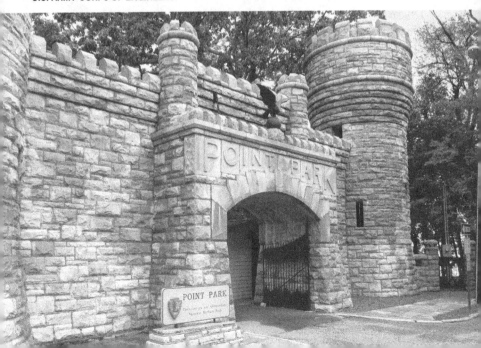

7

Sunset Rock Loop

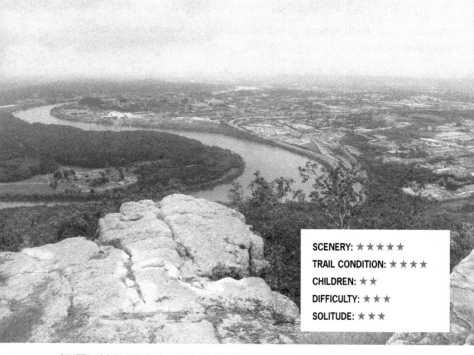

SCENERY: ★ ★ ★ ★ ★
TRAIL CONDITION: ★ ★ ★ ★
CHILDREN: ★ ★
DIFFICULTY: ★ ★ ★
SOLITUDE: ★ ★ ★

CHATTANOOGA AND THE BENDS OF THE TENNESSEE RIVER AS SEEN FROM THE
TOP OF LOOKOUT MOUNTAIN

GPS TRAILHEAD COORDINATES: N35° 00.590' W85° 20.626'

DISTANCE & CONFIGURATION: 4.8-mile balloon

HIKING TIME: 3 hours

HIGHLIGHTS: Views galore, Civil War history

ELEVATION: 2,110' at trailhead, 1,290' at low point

ACCESS: Entrance fee required

MAPS: *Lookout Mountain Trail Map;* USGS *Chattanooga*

FACILITIES: Visitor center, restrooms, picnic area at trailhead

WHEELCHAIR ACCESS: On upper part of Point Park

CONTACTS: Chickamauga & Chattanooga National Military Park, 706-866-9241, nps.gov/chch

Overview

Start your hike atop Lookout Mountain, at Point Park. Grab dramatic vistas from sandstone peninsulas, then cruise along rock bluffs displaying a treasure of geological forms, from rock houses (natural rock shelters) to sandstone walls and boulder gardens. Soak in views beyond the mountain. Stop at Sunset Rock, a superlative rock cliff, to enjoy more panoramas. From there, drop by Gum Spring, then loop your way along the side slope of Lookout, visiting Civil War rifle pits. Climb back to Point Park, regaining 900 feet lost on the descent.

Route Details

This hike combines the drama of Point Park with the natural beauty found on Lookout Mountain in places like Sunset Rock and Gum Spring. Before you enter the impressive stone entrance of Point Park, wander through the visitor center to learn more about the import of Lookout Mountain in Chattanooga's Civil War history. After entering Point Park, join a stone slab path downhill. An asphalt loop curves along the east and west brows of the mountain. Cannon emplacements make for theatrical vistas of the lands below. At the bottom of the green space, take the steps leading down toward Ochs Museum, set on a rock outcrop, with perhaps the finest views anywhere in the region.

Soak up interpretive information in the small stone museum after taking in those awesome views. Below, Moccasin Bend makes its curve. The wooded Cumberland Plateau builds to the northwest. The city of Chattanooga stretches across the riverside flats and beyond. Leave the view and drop down metal stairs, bypassing a sheer bluff that Union soldiers scaled using handmade ladders back in 1863. Note the plaque inlaid in this stone wall to commemorate Pennsylvania soldiers

Turn left near the plaque, joining the Bluff Trail, heading southwest toward Sunset Rock. The mostly level track stretches along the base of stupendous rock ramparts, rising high overhead, pocked with rock shelters. Don't forget to look beyond toward Lookout Valley.

Sunset Rock Loop

At 0.4 mile Rock Springs stands in a cliff alcove on your left. Ahead, walk past stone castles and other fanciful stone constructs. At 0.8 mile come to the Cravens House Trail. It will be your return route. Stay left here with the Bluff

Trail. The rocky highlights continue astride the mostly level path, including disjointed stone pillars rising among the trees. The cliff becomes so precipitous that metal cables have been installed to help keep hikers on the path. Occasional intermittent streams flow across the trail. Watch for stone construction from the Civilian Conservation Corps (CCC) days, including abandoned spurs that head onto rock promontories or simply places where the trail was built up to battle erosion. At 1.2 miles come to a conspicuous rock overhang and fallen boulder. At 1.3 miles the path curves into a wooded watershed. More rock overhangs stand ahead. This is a popular rock climbing area.

At 1.4 miles take the spur left uphill toward Sunset Rock. Stone steps lead to the sandstone promontory. Views open but continue to the rock slab posted with interpretive information—this is THE Sunset Rock. One-hundred-eighty-degree views open toward the west. Wow! Like other Lookout Mountain prominences, this view played a part in strategizing during the Civil War. Other Sunset Rock visitors may have come from the short trail leading from West Brow Road to the rock. Our hike backtracks to the Bluff Trail, continuing south for just a short distance to reach another intersection at 1.6 miles. Here, turn sharply right and downhill, joining the Gum Spring Trail. Descend steep woods, using occasional switchbacks. Pass rocked-in Gum Spring to the right of the trail at 2 miles. Follow alongside the outflow of Gum Spring to reach the Upper Truck Trail at 2.2 miles. Turn right here, crossing the outflow of Gum Spring, then meet the Lower Gum Spring Trail. Stay straight with the Upper Truck Trail, walking a wide and easy path, now at your lowest elevation. At 2.3 miles the Guild Trail leaves left. Pass the site of the CCC camp that operated here in the 1930s before joining the Rifle Pits Trail at 2.7 miles.

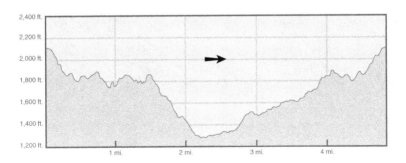

Begin your slow but sure ascent toward Point Park, shaded by dogwoods. At 3.1 miles come to the stonework of the rifle pits. Work around the point of Lookout Mountain to meet the Cravens House Trail at 3.3 miles. Turn sharply right here, rising along the mountain slope. At 4 miles complete the Cravens House Trail. Turn left here on the Bluff Trail and backtrack to the Point Park visitor center. Make sure to visit both bluffs atop Point Park on your return.

Nearby Attractions

The greater Lookout Mountain part of the national battlefield has miles of trails on public lands extending on the east and west sides of Lookout Mountain, even into Georgia.

Directions

From Exit 175 on I-24 west of downtown Chattanooga, take Browns Ferry Road south 0.4 mile to a traffic light and Cummings Highway/US 41/64/11/72. Turn left on Cummings Highway and follow it 0.8 mile to turn right on Alford Hill Drive. Follow Alford Hill Drive to soon reach Old Wauhatchie Pike/TN 318. Turn left on Old Wauhatchie Pike and follow it 1.4 miles to reach TN 148/ Scenic Highway. Turn right on Scenic Highway and follow it 2.3 miles, then veer sharply right on East Brow Road (look for signs to Point Park). Follow East Brow Road 1.1 miles to reach Point Park. Parking is on your left just after curving left past the stone Point Park entrance.

8

Little Cedar Mountain Hike

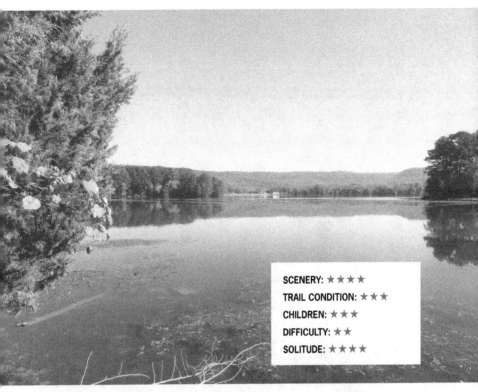

SCENERY: ★ ★ ★ ★
TRAIL CONDITION: ★ ★ ★
CHILDREN: ★ ★ ★
DIFFICULTY: ★ ★
SOLITUDE: ★ ★ ★ ★

SOAK IN THIS VIEW OF NICKAJACK LAKE FROM THE LITTLE CEDAR MOUNTAIN TRAIL.

GPS TRAILHEAD COORDINATES: N35° 01.845' W85° 34.888'

DISTANCE & CONFIGURATION: 3.3-mile balloon

HIKING TIME: 1.8 hours

HIGHLIGHTS: Lake views, limestone outcrops, stone fences

ELEVATION: 700' at trailhead, 895' at high point

ACCESS: No fees, permits, or passes required

MAPS: TVA *Little Cedar Mountain Trail, Nickajack Reservoir;* USGS *Sequatchie TN*

FACILITIES: None

WHEELCHAIR ACCESS: First 100 feet of trail

CONTACTS: Tennessee Valley Authority, 865-632-2101, tva.com

Little Cedar Mountain Hike

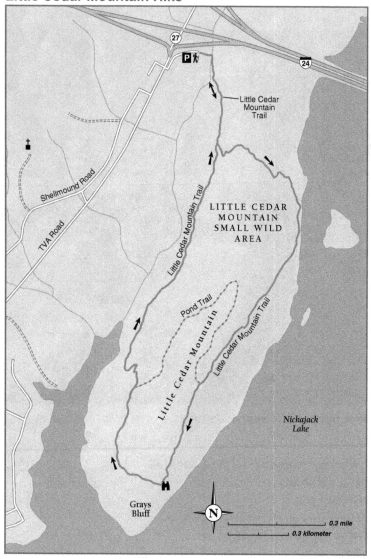

Overview

This fun little hike loops along a ridge, named Little Cedar Mountain, that abuts Nickajack Lake. The trek explores the limestone underpinnings of the mountain, leads through rock gardens, along the lakeshore, and up to bluffs overlooking the mountain-rimmed reservoir. The balance of the circuit hike leads under a forest of cedar and hickory associated with limestone outcroppings.

Route Details

Little Cedar Mountain Small Wild Area is a 320-acre tract along the shores of Nickajack Lake. Before the erection of Hales Bar Dam, later replaced by Nickajack Dam, Little Cedar Mountain was touched by water only at Grays Bluff, rising from the Tennessee River. The mount was bordered by hardscrabble farms growing corn, garden vegetables, and tobacco on limestone-underlain land pocked with sinkholes. The rising waters of Nickajack Lake inundated these farms and other lands, surrounding Little Cedar Mountain on three sides with water in the process.

In creating the chain of lakes to control flooding and generate hydropower on the Tennessee River, Tennessee Valley Authority (TVA) purchased vast tracks of land by eminent domain, flooding one community after another. Part of the land they purchased became shoreline, such as happened to Little Cedar Mountain. TVA decided to preserve this particular tract, underlain by limestone that harbors a special plant community where cedars, hickories, and redbuds thrive, along with scrub oaks and wildflowers, including Beck's leafcup, blazing star, and hoary puccoon. Cedar glades form where the soil is thin and rocky, allowing only specialized plants to survive.

The hike leaves the trailhead kiosk, tracing the asphalt Little Cedar Mountain (LCM) Trail into woods, reaching a bridge spanning a drainage flowing off nearby Anderson Ridge. Speaking of nearby, I-24 is close here, and noisy vehicles

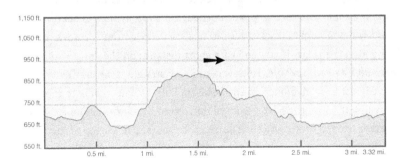

are whizzing by. However, the now natural-surface trail leads south away from the superhighway, tracing the drainage as a singletrack footpath winding under hardwoods and pines. At 0.3 mile you reach the loop portion of the hike. Here, head left, entering rock gardens of emergent limestone. Hickories and cedars, as well as scrub oaks, thrive in less rocky areas. The path is stony to the extreme but winds between the rocks as much as possible. Moss and ferns propagate on the shady sides of the limestone. Look for sinkholes in this karst terrain, a land of rock fissures and an underground plumbing system that leaves most surface streams high and dry save for after rains.

Reach the crest of Little Cedar Mountain in a gap at 0.5 mile. Descend through the stony maze, reaching flats on the east side of the mountain. Here, come along a stone fence, a relic from subsistence farm days, and keep an eye out for other relics from that time. The path now turns south and comes to the shoreline of Nickajack Lake at 0.8 mile. Here, you can look across the water at Sand Mountain, rising 900 feet above the water. To your left extend the shallows of Rankin Cove. As you look out on Rankin Cove, realize it is but one small segment of this reservoir. The impoundment stretches 46 miles up the river valley, covering 10,370 surface acres bordered by more than 179 miles of shoreline. This part of the lake is bordered by Cedar Mountain, Raccoon Mountain, and Sand Mountain. From this viewpoint you can look south into Georgia. Alabama is barely out of sight to the west, as is Nickajack Dam. The energy-producing barrier also has locks for barges and personal craft to link Nickajack to Guntersville Lake downstream. I've personally boated the entire Tennessee River from Knoxville to its end at the Ohio River and pronounce it a first-rate adventure.

But back to our little hiking adventure. Continue south beyond the lake view, rising among the rock maze back to the crest of Little Cedar Mountain, climbing about 250 feet. Top out in wooded, less rocky flats to soon meet the Pond Trail at 1.4 miles. This path shortcuts the main loop and passes a part-time pond atop the ridge. If you go just a short distance on the Pond Trail you can peer into a deep sinkhole. However, you stay straight, still southbound along the edge of a wooded bluff on the LCM Trail. At 1.7 miles come to the edge of Grays Bluff. Here, the partly wooded outcrop reveals far-reaching views to the north, east, and south, as well as down to the lake and to the top of surrounding ridges. Multiple views open in a short distance.

Leave Grays Bluff and its views and reenter rocky woods, curving to the west side of Little Cedar Mountain. Next, wind your way north among limestone rock gardens. At 2.1 miles the other end of the Pond Trail comes in on your right. From there, LCM Trail descends by switchbacks before resuming northbound. Look for the head of a watery cove through the trees to your left. Dip to the base of the mountain in less rocky woods before completing the loop portion of the hike at 3 miles. From here it is a 0.3-mile backtrack to the trailhead.

Nearby Attractions

Nearby Marion County Park is set on Nickajack Lake and offers boating access and campsites year-round. For more information, visit marioncountypark.com.

Directions

From Chattanooga, take I-24 west to Exit 158, Powells Crossroads/TN 27. Exit the interstate and turn left (south) under the interstate. After 0.2 mile turn left onto the signed TVA access road and follow it a short distance to the signed LCM trailhead and parking area.

9 Pot Point Nature Trail

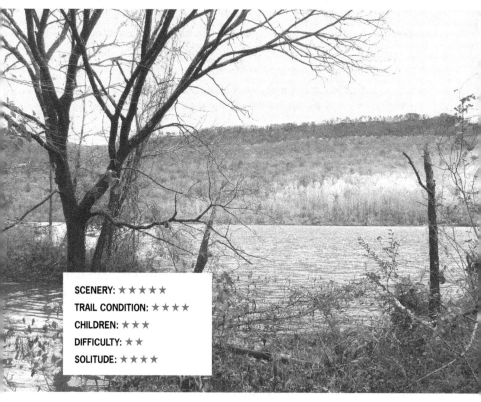

SCENERY: ★ ★ ★ ★ ★
TRAIL CONDITION: ★ ★ ★ ★
CHILDREN: ★ ★ ★
DIFFICULTY: ★ ★
SOLITUDE: ★ ★ ★ ★

VIEW OF THE TENNESSEE RIVER AS IT CUTS THROUGH THE CUMBERLAND PLATEAU

GPS TRAILHEAD COORDINATES: N35° 05.361' W85° 23.948'

DISTANCE & CONFIGURATION: 3.5-mile loop

HIKING TIME: 2 hours

HIGHLIGHTS: Interpretive information, waterside views of Tennessee River and gorge

ELEVATION: 680' at trailhead, 1,080' at high point

ACCESS: No fees, permits, or passes required

MAPS: *Pot Point Nature Trail;* USGS *Wauhatchie*

FACILITIES: None

WHEELCHAIR ACCESS: None

CONTACTS: Tennessee River Gorge Trust, 423-266-0314, trgt.org

Overview

This hike has two distinct segments. The first part explores the lower slope of the Tennessee River Gorge as a self-guided nature trail. Numbered posts accompany a handout detailing human and natural history of the canyon. The second part of the hike dips to the Tennessee River and runs along Chattanooga's master waterway, giving you views of the river, framed by the desiccated tableland through which it cuts.

Route Details

The Tennessee River Gorge Trust is an organization dedicated to preserving the natural components of the 27-mile-long canyon extending from just west of Chattanooga beyond to Nickajack Lake. This trail travels over land purchased by the trust and is an example of private citizens banding together to preserve the natural beauty of the greater Chattanooga area. You can help by joining this organization. To best enjoy this hike, go to the Tennessee River Gorge Trust website and download the self-guided nature trail pamphlet, listed under Pot Point Cabin. Numbered posts correspond to the pamphlet, and you can enjoy the interpretive information included therein.

Pass the trailhead kiosk and immediately enter thick woods on a slender path. Find the first marked interpretive post right off the bat. These posts are intermittently placed throughout the first half of the hike. River Canyon Road runs to your left. Begin hiking beneath sweetgum, red oaks, beech, and other hardwoods. You'll cross the first of many stony wet-weather drainages flowing from the top of the Cumberland Plateau above. Rocks, boulders, and nuggets of all shapes and sizes litter the sloped forest floor, having tumbled from the stony heights. The piled rocks you see are remnants from when this riverside land was tilled or otherwise used as pasturage. Not that the land was particularly alluring; proximity to the Tennessee River was the source of its appeal to farmers of yesteryear, for the grand waterway was a major transportation venue before the land was overlain with the highways we have today. Additionally, the river through the gorge was once infamous for wrecking wooden boats used during the pioneering days of early America. Upon entering the canyon the Tennessee narrowed and became a menacing flow, bounding through the Cumberland Plateau.

Pot Point Nature Trail

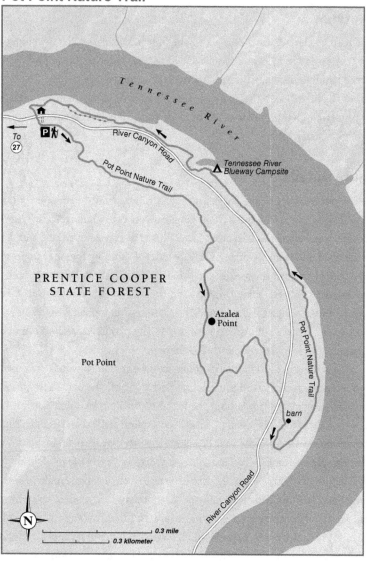

It is placid now that the river has been dammed throughout its length. However, before the Tennessee Valley Authority, the river was subject to floods and had dangerous rapids. Just below you was "the Suck," a terrorizing whirlpool located where Suck Creek met the Tennessee River. If you made it past that, Suck Shoals awaited. Cherokee Indians often ambushed boats as they passed through the gorge. Boatmen were always happy to exit the canyon several miles downstream.

Climb in fits and starts away from the river. The forest is gorgeous here. At 0.5 mile level off, joining an old wagon track. Note the rock walls used to level the lower side of the path here. Resume your climb and reach Azalea Point at 0.9 mile. Toward the end of April this spot blooms brightly. Ahead, come to a level area and you have topped out. Watch for big boulders and scree slopes on the upper end of this flat. The actual Pot Point is far above on the plateau.

At 1.1 miles the trail leaves the flat, picking up a wide track and turning downhill. Begin winding your way among rocky woods on a gentle trail. Come to and cross River Canyon Road at 1.6 miles. Pot Point Nature Trail descends toward bottomland. Come to an old barn at 1.7 miles. This is another relic of days gone by, a time when the river moved faster but riverside life moved slower. Pick up a mown grass track heading right and away from the barn. Soon curve toward the Tennessee. Hike north into wooded flats, full of young gnarly, viny plants, along with ash, hackberry, and tulip trees. This is one of the few trails you can hike on such a big river in a natural setting. Enjoy this, but be apprised these bottoms can be a bit sloppy in spring or after rains.

At 2.3 miles come directly alongside the Tennessee River. Soak in some gorgeous water-level scenes, the river flowing under wooded mountainsides rising to sheer clifflines 1,000 feet above. Look for navigational buoys in the river. During the warm season you may hear or see recreational boaters, but in winter the river is mostly silent. Multiple views keep luring you to the water's edge, despite occasional bits of trash being washed ashore from upstream.

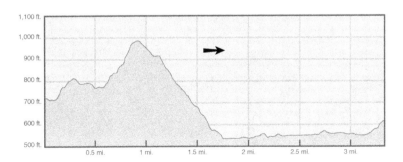

At 2.7 miles the trail opens onto a grassy flat. This is a campsite, part of the Tennessee River Blueway. The trail now circles around a cove and returns to the water's edge. At 3 miles open onto a flat. Here, the trail splits. Stay along the river, as another mown track makes a loop. This minicircuit is part of a butterfly observation trail. The trail leads behind the land trust cabin. Come near the back door of the Pot Point Cabin rental facility before emerging onto River Canyon Road at 3.4 miles, finishing the hike.

Nearby Attractions

The Pot Point Cabin, which you will pass at the end of the hike, is available for day or overnight rental. It can sleep 10 people and accommodates 50 for events. For more information, visit the Tennessee River Gorge Trust website.

Directions

From Chattanooga, take US 27 to the base of Signal Mountain and the junction of US 27 and US 127 northwest of Chattanooga. Take US 127 north 1.6 miles to TN 27. Turn left (west) on TN 27 and follow it 4 miles to River Canyon Road, just before turning into the Suck Creek Gorge. Turn left on River Canyon Road and follow it 4.2 miles. Look right and turn into the Pot Point Biological Field Station. After pulling in, the trailhead is on your left and parking is on your right.

10 Ritchie Hollow Trail to Blowing Wind Falls

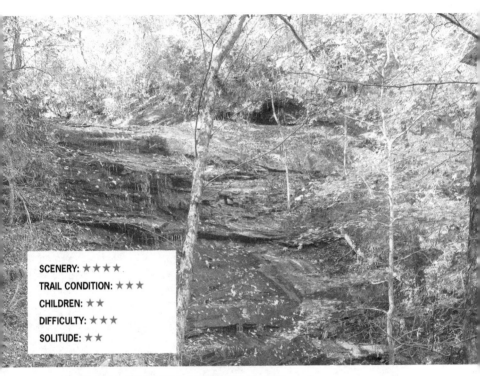

SCENERY: ★ ★ ★ ★

TRAIL CONDITION: ★ ★ ★

CHILDREN: ★ ★

DIFFICULTY: ★ ★ ★

SOLITUDE: ★ ★

BLOWING WIND FALLS CAN SLOW TO A TRICKLE IN AUTUMN.

GPS TRAILHEAD COORDINATES: N35° 05.361' W85° 23.948'

DISTANCE & CONFIGURATION: 3-mile out-and-back

HIKING TIME: 1.6 hours

HIGHLIGHTS: Blowing Wind Falls, lesser cascades, big trees

ELEVATION: 668' at trailhead, 1,262' at high point

ACCESS: No fees, permits, or passes required

MAPS: TRGT *Ritchie Hollow Trail;* USGS *Wauhatchie*

FACILITIES: None

WHEELCHAIR ACCESS: None

CONTACTS: Tennessee River Gorge Trust, 423-266-0314, trgt.org

Ritchie Hollow Trail to Blowing Wind Falls

Overview

The Ritchie Hollow Trail starts at the base of the gorge of the Tennessee River, then cruises along the lower slopes of Walden Ridge, under deep woods and past steep stony vales of Prentice Cooper State Forest to enter Ritchie Hollow. Climb to a cliffline, where 30-foot Blowing Wind Falls spills over an angled ledge into a stone amphitheater with nearby rock houses.

Route Details

This hike traverses the slopes of the Tennessee River Gorge, on a tract that the Tennessee River Gorge Trust had a hand in protecting. Working with landowners, as well as state organizations, the trust continues to try to keep the 27-mile-long Grand Canyon of the Tennessee in its natural state. And you will enjoy beauty aplenty on this trek, including big trees among big boulders, steep stony hollows with tumbling cascades, and the cliffs of Walden Ridge, from which Blowing Wind Falls makes its tumble.

The Ritchie Hollow Trail, opened in 2018, is your conduit to reach Blowing Wind Falls. This newer trail links the Tennessee River Gorge Trust trailhead with the Cumberland Trail atop Walden Ridge. The upper end of the Ritchie Hollow Trail ends at Davis Pond, an auto-accessible campsite on the crest of the mountain. Important note: Check the Prentice Cooper State Forest website for hunt dates, as this trail is closed during that time.

From the parking area—also shared with the Pot Point Nature Trail—with your back to the Tennessee River, head right and uphill on a gravel doubletrack to find a trail signboard at the edge of the woods. Here, you join the singletrack Ritchie Hollow Trail as it travels westerly along the lower slope of Walden Ridge. The Tennessee River can be seen through the trees to your right, and Raccoon Mountain rises 1,200 feet across the water, forming the other side of the Tennessee River Gorge. The trail undulates along the slope under a tall mantle of

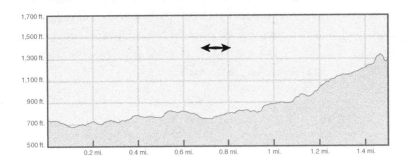

beech, sycamore, and oak trees undergirded with ferns. The trail doesn't always go where you think it will or should go. It is obviously taking the scenic route, as is evidenced by the huge beech tree you pass at 0.1 mile.

At 0.3 mile the Ritchie Hollow Trail leads you into interestingly named Chestnut Bridge Hollow. Here, a rock-strewn stream enters the hollow, sporting tiered cascades both above and below the creek crossing. Rocks, as well as a short stone bridge, have been placed to aid a dry-footed passage, but most of the time you won't need help, as the creek is usually low. Curve back out to the slope, working around sizable boulders.

At 0.6 mile turn into the hollow of Blowing Springs Branch. This smallish stream also has pretty little cascades but is not Blowing Wind Falls. I don't understand why the namer of the waterfall used part of the name of a nearby stream to give Blowing Wind Falls a moniker. Name aside, the Ritchie Hollow Trail continues its westerly ways, still not climbing. At 1 mile you are on a relatively level area rich with tulip trees. The easy hiking is over as you start ascending by switchbacks and turning toward more desiccated Ritchie Hollow. The slope of the mountain steepens. Cliffs rise above you. By 1.4 miles you have picked up a rough old jeep track and are following it among mountain laurel and rhododendron. Shortly ahead look for a sign indicating a spur trail to WATER-FALL. Take this path right, descending into a stony amphitheater, traveling along an overhanging cliffline. At the base of the stony amphitheater stands Blowing Wind Falls, spilling 30 feet in a widening, tiered sheet over a layered stone wall, angled outward. A clear, shallow pool forms along with sand and rock at the base of the cataract. This low-volume spiller is best enjoyed from winter through spring. By summer—barring thunderstorms—it often barely dribbles over its rock face and, despite being framed by the bright colors of autumn, can nearly dry up during that season. Boulders at the base of the falls make for fine waterfall admiration seating. In addition to the cataract, you can look up to your left to see some small rock houses and a columnar arch. Enjoy the setting and the cataract before backtracking to the trailhead.

Nearby Attractions

The Pot Point Cabin, near the trailhead, is available for day or overnight rental. It can sleep 10 people and accompany 50 for events. For more information, visit the Tennessee River Gorge Trust website.

Directions

From Chattanooga, take US 27 to the base of Signal Mountain and the junction of US 27 and US 127 northwest of Chattanooga. Take US 127 north 1.6 miles to TN 27. Turn left (west) on TN 27 and follow it 4 miles to River Canyon Road, just before turning into the Suck Creek Gorge. Turn left on River Canyon Road and follow it 4.2 miles. Look right and turn into the Pot Point Biological Field Station. After you pull in, the parking is on your right, and the Ritchie Hollow Trail can be accessed uphill from the parking area.

PICTURESQUE BEECH TREES GRACE THE TRAILSIDE WOODS.

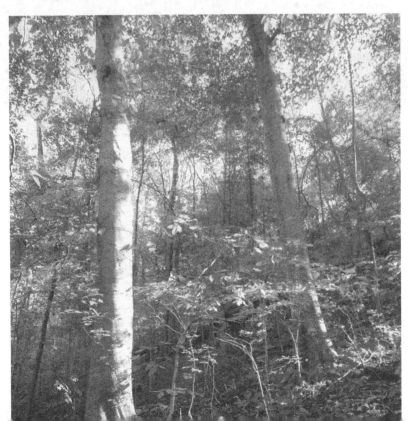

Snoopers Rock
Natural Bridge Hike

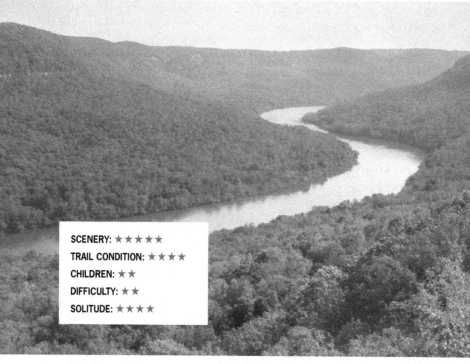

SCENERY: ★ ★ ★ ★ ★
TRAIL CONDITION: ★ ★ ★ ★
CHILDREN: ★ ★
DIFFICULTY: ★ ★
SOLITUDE: ★ ★ ★ ★

SNOOPERS ROCK PRESENTS A FIRST-RATE VIEW INTO THE GRAND CANYON OF THE TENNESSEE RIVER.

GPS TRAILHEAD COORDINATES: N35° 06.075' W85° 25.732'

DISTANCE & CONFIGURATION: 6-mile out-and-back

HIKING TIME: 3.5 hours

HIGHLIGHTS: Incredible view, rock arch

ELEVATION: 1,600' at trailhead, 1,760' at high point

ACCESS: No fees, permits, or passes required

MAPS: *Cumberland Trail—Tennessee River Gorge, Prentice Cooper State Forest Hiking Trail Map;* USGS *Wauhatchie*

FACILITIES: Picnic tables, restroom

WHEELCHAIR ACCESS: None

CONTACTS: Justin P. Wilson Cumberland Trail State Park, 423-566-2229, tnstateparks.com; Prentice Cooper State Forest, 423-658-5551, tn.gov/agriculture/forests.html

Overview

This hike visits a portion of the Grand Canyon of Tennessee, where the Tennessee River cuts a 1,000-foot gorge through the Cumberland Plateau. Within the confines of large and wild Prentice Cooper State Forest, you will first come to the large, wide, and top-notch vista at Snoopers Rock, where river gorge panoramas amaze. You will then pick up the Cumberland Trail, hiking the canyon rim and the stream valleys that cut their own chasms, eventually reaching Natural Bridge, a sturdy stone arch over which you hike.

Route Details

Note: The state forest is closed to hikers during certain spring and fall hunt dates. Check ahead for these weekends before you drive to the trailhead. The dates are posted on the state forest website.

This hike uses part of what is known as the Pot Point Trail. Leave the parking area on a white-blazed connector trail that leads left, easterly, from behind the trailhead kiosk. Take this singletrack path downhill, rambling through hardwoods to quickly pass a small pond. Come along a small branch and reach a trail junction at 0.3 mile. Here, you meet the Cumberland Trail. The way to Natural Bridge turns right here; however, keep straight and walk past the northbound Cumberland Trail before opening onto the expansive flat stone of Snoopers Rock. The views are inspiring. The Grand Canyon of the Tennessee River stretches both north and south as it bends out of sight, bordered by high bluffs dropping to steep wooded slopes that fall to the waterway. Raccoon Mountain stands boldly across the river. The wide-open rock slab is about as fine of an overlook as there is.

Backtrack to the southbound Cumberland Trail and head toward Natural Bridge. Work your way out to the gorge rim. Look back toward the pale stone of Snoopers Rock jutting into the canyon. Turn into Muddy Branch Hollow, crossing normally clear Muddy Branch at 0.5 mile. Pay attention here as the trail goes on and off a steep roadbed. Climb back toward the canyon rim in oak-dominated woods. It's a long way down from here—1,000 feet to the river! The terrain is difficult, extremely sloped and rocky. Walking the path can be a challenge; building it must've been tough. Make a hard switchback to the right at 0.9 mile, then level off and resume your southbound ways. Rock outcrops are abundant.

Snoopers Rock Natural Bridge Hike

Turn into Ritchie Hollow, one of the larger coves in this gorge, at 1.2 miles. Hike a mountainside flat, with outcrops and rock houses (natural rock shelters) aplenty above you. Cross the first major tributary of Ritchie Hollow at 1.6 miles, then pass the intersection with the Ritchie Hollow Trail before bridging two more tributaries at 2.1 and 2.2 miles. The path is quite stony in spots. Curve back toward the Tennessee River, reaching the canyon rim at 2.8 miles. Cruise the edge of the gulf. Wintertime views are extensive along this wooded rim. If I had to be a tree, I would want to be one of these sturdy oaks perched here, along the brow of the canyon. At 3.1 miles, a narrow trail connecting to a rock slab lures you left. The views are only partial though, and they don't even compare to those of Snoopers Rock.

This overlook immediately precedes the Natural Bridge. You will walk atop the Natural Bridge first. Casual hikers might not even notice that they are using a stone walkway over an opening below. However, the Natural Bridge is signed. It's not too hard to drop off the trail and get under the arch. Down here you can appreciate the stone span that extends about 20 feet high and 40 feet wide—a squat, sturdy conduit.

This arch is a by-product of the erosive process. Arches can be formed in numerous ways, including more violent, instantaneous means, such as rock collapse, versus unhurried erosion by water. Arches have their own special terminology. The span of rock over which you walk, the actual natural bridge, is called a lintel. The flat part of this bridge, in this case, where the trail travels, is called the deck. From below you can look up at the span of the arch. This span is the widest distance between the two arch pillars. The clearance is the highest point of the arch down to the ground.

Natural Bridge is but one of many highlights located within 25,000-acre Prentice Cooper State Forest. The preserve, named for a Tennessee governor, was established in 1945, after the state bought subsistence farms, pasturage, and forestland here on the plateau. It was once a hunting ground of the Cherokee

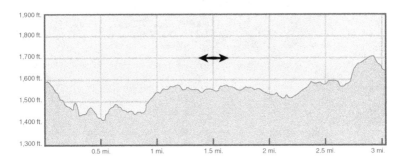

Indians, who lived along the Tennessee River where Chattanooga now lies. Today, the state land is managed for forestry and hunting, but it also has one of the most spectacular sections of the Cumberland Trail, part of which this hike covers.

Nearby Attractions

Campers can use several trail-accessible backcountry campsites in the forest, or car camp at Davis Pond or at the state forest entrance. Camping conditions are primitive.

Directions

From Chattanooga, take US 27 to the base of Signal Mountain and the junction of US 27 and US 127 northwest of Chattanooga. Take US 127 north 1.6 miles to TN 27. Turn left (west) on TN 27 and follow it 8 miles to Choctaw Trail and a sign for Prentice Cooper Wildlife Management Area. Turn left on Choctaw Trail and follow it 0.2 mile to reach Game Reserve Road. Turn left on Game Reserve Road and enter Prentice Cooper State Forest, where it becomes Tower Road. Keep forward on gravel Tower Road 4.6 miles to the Cumberland Trail parking area on your left.

Overlooks of Mullens Cove and Ransom Hollow

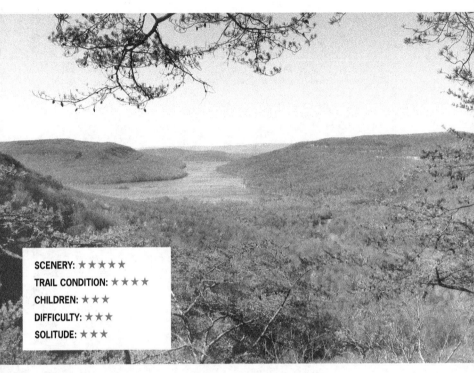

SCENERY: ★★★★★
TRAIL CONDITION: ★★★★
CHILDREN: ★★★
DIFFICULTY: ★★★
SOLITUDE: ★★★

RANSOM HOLLOW IS ONE OF MY FAVORITE OVERLOOKS IN THE SOUTHEAST.

GPS TRAILHEAD COORDINATES: N35° 06.075' W85° 25.732'

DISTANCE & CONFIGURATION: 4.7-mile out-and-back

HIKING TIME: 3 hours

HIGHLIGHTS: Dual vistas, river gorge

ELEVATION: 1,600' at trailhead, 1,660' at high point

ACCESS: No fees, permits, or passes required

MAPS: *Cumberland Trail—Tennessee River Gorge, Prentice Cooper State Forest Hiking Trail Map;* USGS *Wauhatchie*

FACILITIES: Picnic tables, restroom

WHEELCHAIR ACCESS: None

CONTACTS: Justin P. Wilson Cumberland Trail State Park, 423-566-2229, tnstateparks.com; Prentice Cooper State Forest, 423-658-5551, tn.gov/agriculture/forests.html

Overlooks of Mullens Cove and Ransom Hollow

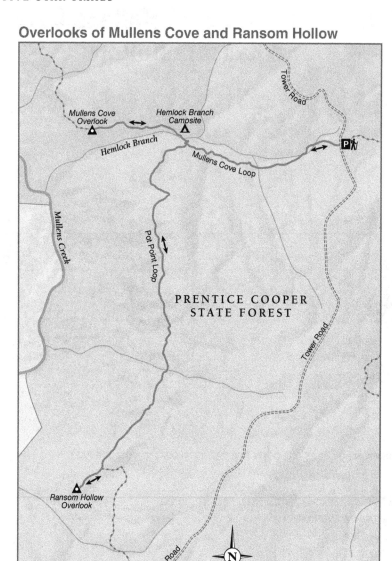

Overview

This trek visits two overlooks straddled on the edge of the Mullens Creek gorge. First, descend along pretty little Hemlock Branch, crossing the clear stream, then head for Mullens Cove Overlook, where the rock-walled gorge of Mullens

Creek opens to the Tennessee River. Backtrack, then head to Ransom Hollow Overlook, where an outcrop presents an extensive sweep of the Grand Canyon of the Tennessee River as far as the eye can see. Elevation changes are minimal, making a narrow rocky trail the main challenge.

Route Details

Note: Prentice Cooper State Forest is closed to hikers during certain spring and fall hunt dates. Check with the state forest for these weekends before you drive to the trailhead. The dates are posted on the state forest website.

From the parking area on the east side of Tower Road, with the picnic area to your left, walk just a few feet farther along Tower Road and look right for the white-blazed Mullens Cove Loop crossing Tower Road. Drop into a shallow hollow, strewn with leaf litter fallen from hardwoods. A streamlet begins forming on your right. Follow it westerly, downhill. This is upper Hemlock Branch. Step over stony tributaries of Hemlock Branch on your descent. Note the preponderance of holly trees here. Mountain laurel and, of course, hemlocks find their place too. Hemlocks of the Cumberland Plateau are in peril. The hemlock woolly adelgid, an Asian bug, has been decimating hemlocks in the East. However, there is hope. Land managers can use two control techniques: spraying the trees with a soapy insecticide that kills only the adelgid or releasing a bug that kills the adelgid. The University of Tennessee is continuing research on this situation.

Reach a trail intersection at 0.6 mile. Hemlock Branch is gurgling among boulders just below. You will return to this intersection later. For now, turn right, descending to rock-hop the stream and reach the Hemlock Branch backcountry

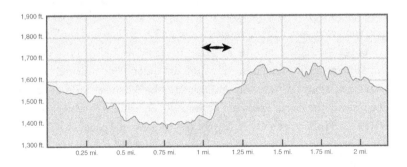

campsite, nestled against the waterway in a small flat. Mullens Cove Loop passes directly through the campsite.

Continue along a rock- and tree-covered slope, while Hemlock Branch dives away, descending in cascades toward Mullens Creek. At 0.7 mile the trail briefly picks up an obvious old roadbed. Turn left, following this route, then split away right, back on a singletrack path. A xeric forest of chestnut oak and pines borders the trail. Reach the signed, short spur trail to the Mullens Cove Overlook at 1 mile. A stone outcrop provides your viewing perch. Before you, the gorge of Mullens Creek widens, ultimately opening to the Tennessee River and beyond. Note the rock walls lining the gorge.

Backtrack to the trail intersection near Hemlock Branch. Now pick up the Pot Point Loop, heading toward Ransom Hollow Overlook. This path is also singletrack. Follow the serpentine trail uphill, curving out of the Hemlock Branch watershed on a steep slope. The terrain briefly levels out and then you head southbound on a slope dropping to Mullens Creek. Wind in and out of small streambeds cutting vertically for the lowlands below. A great oak forest shades the path.

Views open through leafless trees. The tan rock walls of the Mullens Creek gorge stand out. At 2.3 miles the trail comes to a hollow littered with gigantic boulders. Initially, it seems the path ends. As you near, the trail simply slices between some of these gray giants, then crosses the stream forming the hollow. Watch for a slide cascade above the creek crossing.

Beyond the boulder squeeze, the trail continues along the rim to reach a trail intersection at 2.6 miles. Here, stay right with the spur trail leading to Ransom Hollow Overlook. This path wanders through a flat before dead-ending at a rock overlook at 2.7 miles. Framed in pines, the panorama opens west. Ransom Hollow opens to your left. You can hear the flowing stream that cuts the hollow. Beyond your perch, the view opens onto Nickajack Lake and the Tennessee River Gorge continuing into the distance. The maw of Mullens Cove opens to your right. Rock walls stand near the mountaintops of ridges near and far. River islands string along the waterway. At this point, the Tennessee River has curved around nearly the entire Prentice Cooper State Forest, effectively creating an elevated island of nature and keeping the resource the wild parcel that it is. This is one of my favorite overlooks in the Southeast. From the overlook it is 2 miles back to the trailhead.

Nearby Attractions

Campers can use several trail-accessible backcountry campsites in the forest or car camp at Davis Pond or at the state forest entrance. Camping conditions are primitive.

Directions

From Chattanooga, take US 27 to the base of Signal Mountain and the junction of US 27 and US 127 northwest of Chattanooga. Take US 127 north 1.6 miles to TN 27. Turn left (west) on TN 27 and follow it 8 miles to Choctaw Trail and a sign for Prentice Cooper Wildlife Management Area. Turn left on Choctaw Trail and follow it 0.2 mile to reach Game Reserve Road. Turn left on Game Reserve Road and enter Prentice Cooper State Forest, where it becomes Tower Road. Keep forward on gravel Tower Road 4.6 miles to the trail parking area on your left.

THE VIEW OF MULLENS COVE HOLDS ITS OWN.

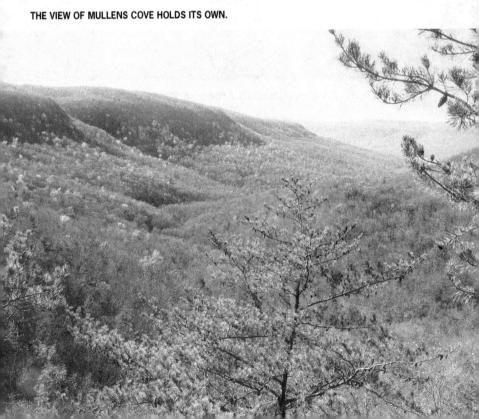

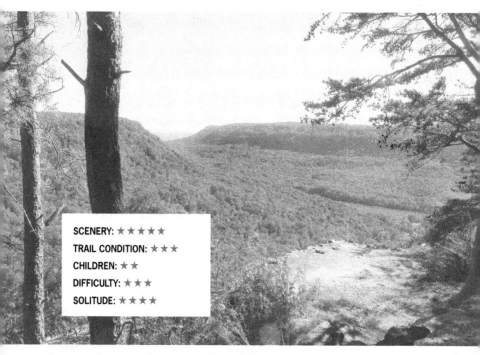

SCENERY: ★ ★ ★ ★ ★
TRAIL CONDITION: ★ ★ ★
CHILDREN: ★ ★
DIFFICULTY: ★ ★ ★
SOLITUDE: ★ ★ ★ ★

THE SUCK CREEK GORGE AND TENNESSEE RIVER OPEN BEFORE LAWSONS ROCK.

GPS TRAILHEAD COORDINATES: N35° 07.960' W85° 25.150'

DISTANCE & CONFIGURATION: 6.4-mile out-and-back

HIKING TIME: 4 hours

HIGHLIGHTS: Indian Rockhouse, Lawsons Rock Overlook, geological wonders

ELEVATION: 1,860' at trailhead, 1,380' at high point

ACCESS: No fees, permits, or passes required

MAPS: *Cumberland Trail—Tennessee River Gorge, Prentice Cooper State Forest Hiking Trail Map;* USGS *Ketner Gap*

FACILITIES: Picnic tables, restroom

WHEELCHAIR ACCESS: None

CONTACTS: Justin P. Wilson Cumberland Trail State Park, 423-566-2229, tnstateparks.com; Prentice Cooper State Forest, 423-658-5551, tn.gov/agriculture/forests.html

Overview

This hike features two major highlights amid everywhere-you-look scenery. First, make a narrow passage between two giant boulders to emerge at the Indian Rockhouse, a large and airy overhang. Head east below the rim of the Tennessee River Gorge, where you will see a plethora of sheer bluffs, rock ramparts, and stone palisades. Turn into the Suck Creek Gorge, with its own geological features, such as spirelike pedestal rocks. Detour away from the rim into Sulphur Creek. Reach the outcrop of Lawsons Rock, where a panorama spreads down the Suck Creek Gorge to the Tennessee River and beyond to Elder Mountain.

Route Details

Note: Prentice Cooper State Forest is closed to hikers during certain spring and fall hunt dates. Check with the state forest for these weekends before you drive to the trailhead. The dates are posted on the state forest website.

This hike is best executed from late fall through early spring, when the leaves are off the trees. This way you can fully appreciate the myriad geological formations along the way. The trailhead parking is on the west side of Tower Road. Cross Tower Road and pick up a singletrack path as it descends southwesterly through white oak woods. Turn south to cross a forest road at 0.3 mile. Your descent sharpens. The drop-off of the Tennessee River Gorge becomes evident ahead. At 0.5 mile turn into a slender stone stairwell, squeezing between two massive gray boulders, a hidden passage off the cliffline. Emerge below the gorge rim to find a trail junction. The Cumberland Trail goes left and right. Walk left and instantly come under the Indian Rockhouse. This tall overhang faces southeast. It surely made for a good wintertime shelter, shielding the cold north winds and precipitation-laden fronts. The shelter floor is very level and dry as well. Interestingly, Tennessee's Cumberland Plateau is dotted with overhangs named Indian Rockhouse, from this one all the way to Pickett State Park near the Kentucky state line.

Hike along the base of a cliffline with rock walls and ample fallen boulders. Occasional streamlets furrow the heavily wooded terrain. Tennessee's Grand Canyon falls away to your right. The river is making a 180-degree bend around

Lawsons Rock via Indian Rockhouse

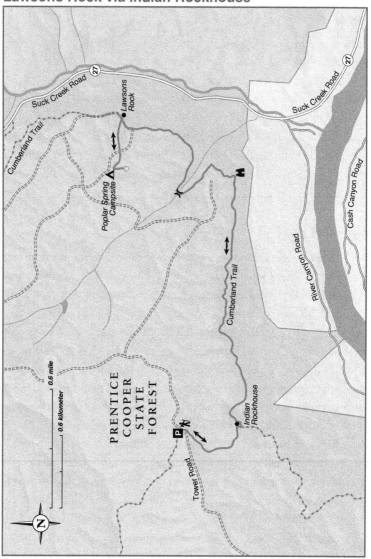

Elder Mountain. The views are breathtaking and are almost continual when the leaves are off the trees. The scenery is so good you can't decide whether to focus on the nearby geology or the far-off vistas outlined by pines clinging to stony precipices. At 1 mile bisect a gas line clearing that opens up views of its own.

Ahead, walk under a brittle cliffline, with rotten layers of rock crumbling downhill. At 1.2 miles you will step over an unnamed streambed that will feature a waterfall in spring. The veil-like drop spills about 12 feet over a rock ledge. Keep looking above the trail—the number of rock houses (natural rock shelters) and cliffs is staggering. The main path, the Cumberland Trail, is in good shape, especially in comparison to the inhospitable terrain through which it travels.

The elevation change has thus far been minimal. At 2 miles curve into the Suck Creek Gorge. Faint trails lead right to rock outcrops that provide good vistas of the confluence of the Tennessee River and Suck Creek far below. The Tennessee River is the largest waterway that cuts through the Cumberland Plateau. Logic mandates that the Tennessee would also cut the deepest and most dramatic gorge through the plateau. And it does.

Beyond the perch, turn into Suck Creek Gorge. Nearby, look for precariously perched slender pedestal rocks, nature's monuments formed by time and erosion. They rise 30 or more feet from the forest floor. Turn into bouldery, cliff-lined Sulphur Branch hollow, bridging the stream at 2.4 miles. Slice through a boulder jumble at 2.8 miles, climbing to a break in the plateau. Emerge on relatively level terrain amid pines, grass, briers, and blueberries. The walking is easy. Reach a four-way trail junction at 3.2 miles. The Cumberland Trail keeps straight. A faint spur trail leads left a quarter mile to the Poplar Springs back-country campsite. The short spur right leads to the gray outcrop of Lawsons Rock. Suck Creek cuts a chasm below. From the open outcrop Signal Mountain stands across the stream. The Grand Canyon of the Tennessee cuts its way around Elder Mountain. If Suck Creek is up, you will hear its roar and be able to see rapids downstream from Lawsons Rock.

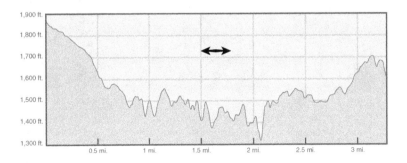

The Poplar Springs campsite access trail crosses a forest road and leads uphill. Another faint, short trail connects the campsite to a wooded ravine and Poplar Springs. On the far side of the spring you will find a circular pit, piled rocks, and metal remains. This was an old moonshine operation that got its water from the spring.

Nearby Attractions

Campers can use several trail-accessible backcountry camping areas in the forest, including Poplar Springs campsite, or car camp at Davis Pond or at the state forest entrance. Camping conditions are primitive.

Directions

From Chattanooga, take US 27 to the base of Signal Mountain and the junction of US 27 and US 127 northwest of Chattanooga. Take US 127 north 1.6 miles to TN 27. Turn left (west) on TN 27 and follow it 8 miles to Choctaw Trail and a sign for Prentice Cooper Wildlife Management Area. Turn left on Choctaw Trail and follow it 0.2 mile to reach Game Reserve Road. Turn left on Game Reserve Road and enter Prentice Cooper State Forest, where it becomes Tower Road. Keep forward on gravel Tower Road 2.6 miles to the Cumberland Trail parking area on your left.

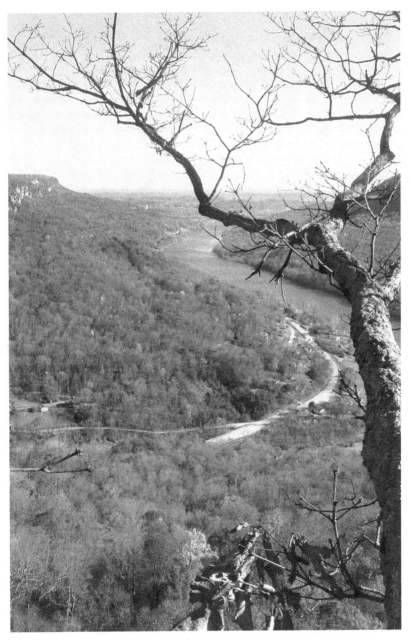

LOOKING THROUGH THE MOUTH OF THE GRAND CANYON OF THE TENNESSEE RIVER

Tennessee Cumberlands (Hikes 14–22)

Tennessee Cumberlands

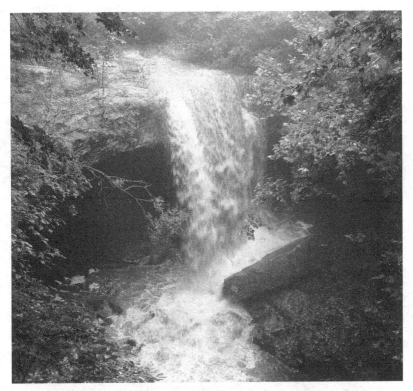

LAUREL FALLS FROTHS FOLLOWING A THUNDERSTORM. (SEE HIKE 17, PAGE 103)

14 Foster Falls Loop

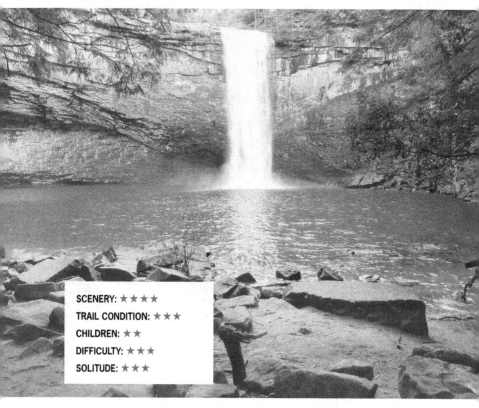

SCENERY: ★ ★ ★ ★
TRAIL CONDITION: ★ ★ ★
CHILDREN: ★ ★
DIFFICULTY: ★ ★ ★
SOLITUDE: ★ ★ ★

FOSTER FALLS AS SEEN FROM THE BASE OF ITS LARGE PLUNGE POOL

GPS TRAILHEAD COORDINATES: N35° 10.943', W85° 40.474'

DISTANCE & CONFIGURATION: 4.6-mile loop with out-and-back

HIKING TIME: 3 hours

HIGHLIGHTS: Waterfall, vistas, climbing bluffs, big pool

ELEVATION: 1,730' at trailhead, 1,600' at low point

ACCESS: No fees, permits, or passes required

MAPS: *South Cumberland State Park—Fiery Gizzard*; USGS *White City*

FACILITIES: Restroom, water, picnic area at trailhead

WHEELCHAIR ACCESS: None

CONTACTS: South Cumberland State Park, 931-924-2980, tnstateparks.com/parks/south-cumberland

Overview

Take the Fiery Gizzard Trail to 60-foot Foster Falls, then walk the rim of Little Gizzard Gulf. Vistas open to the deeply carved valley where rock bluffs contrast forested hills. Reach Laurel Branch Overlook, one of many vistas, also passing rain-dependent waterfalls diving into the gorge below. Backtrack, then make a rugged loop below the gorge rim. Reach the large plunge pool and the base of Foster Falls for yet another view of the cascade before finishing the hike.

Route Details

This hike primarily uses the Fiery Gizzard Trail to explore what was formerly Foster Falls Small Wild Area, which was owned by the Tennessee Valley Authority but has since been conferred to the state of Tennessee and incorporated into greater South Cumberland State Park, an agglomeration of wild tracts in this area. The term *gulf* is commonly used by residents of the Cumberland Plateau to describe gorges. The other part of this unusual name—Fiery Gizzard—was purportedly given to the valley by Daniel Boone after he burned his dinner over a campfire hereabouts. The hike's first part is quite easy, as you ride the rim of Fiery Gizzard Gulf. However, hiking below the gorge rim means irregular terrain, but you can avoid this by simply making an out-and-back hike and skipping the below-rim loop.

At the trailhead, walk toward the picnic shelter, passing a sign-in registration and kiosk. Join the Fiery Gizzard Trail, angling right along the power line. Foster Falls rumbles nearby. Dip to bridge Little Gizzard Creek a short piece above Foster Falls. Magnolia, holly, hemlock, and mountain laurel shade the rocky stream.

Climb away from Little Gizzard Creek into hickory-oak hardwoods. At 0.3 mile a spur trail leaves right to Father Adamz Campground, primarily used by rock climbers and Friday night backpacker late arrivals. Hike astride the Little Gizzard Creek gorge, coming to the rocky overlook of Foster Falls at 0.5 mile. The 60-foot torrent dives from a sheer rock rim, then crashes into a huge plunge pool. Note the circular amphitheater of rock over which the watercourse tumbles.

Continue beyond the overlook. Hemlocks and holly add an evergreen touch to the upland hardwoods. Pines are most prevalent along the edge of the

Foster Falls Loop

gulf and at times will have a grassy understory. At 0.6 mile pass the second spur trail to Father Adamz Campground. Curve past mossy wet areas that will have boardwalks. Watch for side trails created by hikers, seeking views along the rim.

At 0.9 mile reach a trail junction. Here, Climbers Access 1 splits left. Keep straight on the Fiery Gizzard Trail to reach Climbers Access 2 at 1.1 miles. This will be your return route, but for now continue on the Fiery Gizzard Trail. The rim walk leads to a bridge and unnamed stream at 1.3 miles. Enjoy a southerly overlook into the main Fiery Gizzard Gulf. The hard-to-see stream spills from the rim and may run dry in late summer or fall. The path wanders through remarkably level woods. Bridge another seasonal stream at 1.8 miles, then reach a rocky vista of the 700-foot-deep gulf.

Continue west into the Laurel Branch gorge. At 2.1 miles a spur trail leads left to an overlook. Just ahead, reach the signed trail into the Small Wilds backcountry camp, a level respite with several sites scattered in the woods. Dip to bridge a tributary, which drops off the rim just below the trail crossing. A user-created trail leads left just beyond the bridge to an overlook, while the main path continues a short distance to a rock outcrop and the Laurel Branch overlook at 2.3 miles. Soak in "gorge-ous" views of vertical stone walls and outcrops shining amid green forests.

From this point return 1.2 miles to Climbers Access 2, which is reached at 3.5 miles. For an easy hike, continue backtracking on the Fiery Gizzard Trail all the way to the trailhead. But for geological wonderment, turn right and take the climbers' access into the gulf. Soon descend the rim by steps, passing a cool rock house (natural rock shelter). Reach the base of the cliff, and head left, watching for tree blazes. Ramble between big boulders beneath a rising steep bluff. At 3.8 miles stone steps lead to a designated climbing area, but the stairwell does not scale the rim. The stony, irregular track is very slow going. Stumble to another junction at 3.9 miles. Here, Climbers Access 1 leads left to reconnect

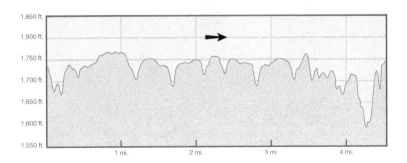

with the Fiery Gizzard Trail. Keep straight, navigating a rocky path bordered by mammoth overhanging rock houses. In wetter times expect drips and seeps flowing from the bluffs above. Also watch for bolted-in carabiners—and maybe rock climbers themselves.

By 4.1 miles you can hear Little Gizzard Creek. The gorge is closing in and hemlocks thicken. Meet a suspension bridge at 4.2 miles. Walk just a short distance to view Foster Falls and its enormous plunge pool from another perspective, then take the suspension bridge over Little Gizzard Creek. From here, climb to the gorge rim. Join a power line cut and turn left, passing a wooden viewpoint of Foster Falls. From there, a wooden boardwalk leads to the trailhead, completing your hike at 4.6 miles.

Nearby Attractions

Foster Falls has a drive-up campground adjacent to the trailhead. It offers 26 sites spread along a loop and makes a fine base camp from which to hike the area. Spacious campsites have concrete picnic tables. The campground is generally open from late March through November.

Directions

From Exit 155 on I-24 west of Chattanooga, take TN 28 north 1.5 miles. Join US 41 north and follow it through Jasper for 9.5 miles to reach Foster Falls Road. Turn left into the park. The official address is 498 Foster Falls Road, Tracy Highway 41, Sequatchie, TN. The trailhead offers restrooms, water, and a covered picnic shelter.

Grundy Forest Day Loop

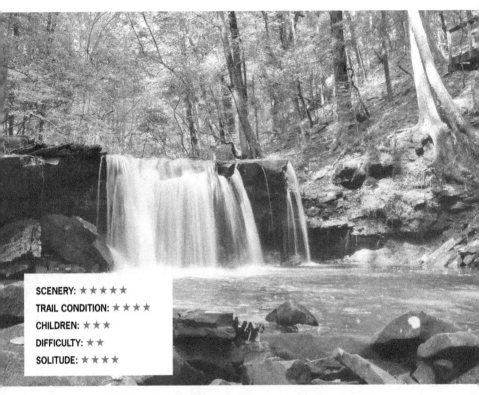

SCENERY: ★ ★ ★ ★ ★
TRAIL CONDITION: ★ ★ ★ ★
CHILDREN: ★ ★ ★
DIFFICULTY: ★ ★
SOLITUDE: ★ ★ ★ ★

HANES HOLE FALLS IS BUT ONE OF SEVERAL CATARACTS ON THIS HIKE.

GPS TRAILHEAD COORDINATES: N35° 15.117' W85° 44.842'

DISTANCE & CONFIGURATION: 3-mile loop with spur

HIKING TIME: 2 hours

HIGHLIGHTS: Giant hemlock, multiple waterfalls, geological wonders, swimming holes

ELEVATION: 1,810' at trailhead, 1,620' at low point

ACCESS: No fees, permits, or passes required

MAPS: *South Cumberland State Park—Fiery Gizzard;* USGS *Tracy City, Burrow Cove, Monteagle*

FACILITIES: Restroom, picnic area at trailhead

WHEELCHAIR ACCESS: None

CONTACTS: South Cumberland State Park, 931-924-2980, tnstateparks.com/parks/south-cumberland

Grundy Forest Day Loop

Overview

Simply stated, Grundy Forest has some of the most concentrated magnificence in the South. From the trailhead, descend to Little Fiery Gizzard Creek and Cave Spring Rock House, complemented by an ancient hemlock. Down valley you will reach Blue Hole Falls and a big swimming hole. Leave the loop to view water-carved Black Canyon just below the confluence of Big and Little Fiery Gizzard Creeks. The Chimney Rocks rise before coming to Sycamore Falls, situated in a scenic flat ideal for natural contemplation. Backtrack, now heading up Big Fiery Gizzard Creek, where Hanes Hole Falls skims off a slickrock slide. Visit an old Civilian Conservation Corps (CCC) camp, now a backcountry campsite. Pass tantalizing Schoolhouse Branch Falls, then reach the trailhead.

Route Details

Picturesque Grundy Forest, a designated Tennessee State Natural Area, was one of the Volunteer State's first preserves. In 1935 residents of Tracy City donated a 212-acre parcel that contains the bulk of the natural features on this hike. Starting from near the picnic shelter, curve left down to Little Fiery Gizzard Creek. The stream slips swiftly and noisily between massive boulders and smaller rocks. At 0.1 mile come to Cave Spring Rock House, an immense overhanging shelter. Cave Spring emerges from the rear of the rock house (natural rock shelter). Note the ancient hemlock, five centuries in the making, guarding the shelter. This tree is being protected from the hemlock woolly adelgid, which is decimating hemlocks in the East. Land managers are using two techniques: spraying the trees with a soapy insecticide that kills only the adelgid and releasing a bug that kills the adelgid. There's not enough money or manpower to rescue all of the Cumberland Plateau's hemlocks, but more will be saved here than in the main Appalachian chain to the east, where the adelgid has spread nearly unchecked.

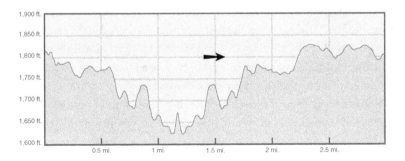

Hike along the fast-moving, evanescent waterway framed in verdant hardwoods and evergreens. Imposing gorge walls, hefty boulders, and other geological formations complement the flora. Trek deeper into the water-carved chasm sporting everywhere-you-look beauty. Shoals are nearly continuous. Schoolhouse Branch comes in on your right at 0.4 mile. Little Fiery Gizzard Creek spills in rockslide cascades at the confluence.

Come to Blue Hole Falls at 0.5 mile. The cataract is named for the opulent opalescent pool below the modest 10-foot falls. Locals have swum here as long as there have been locals. Ahead, the narrow, root-laced trail cuts deeper into the mossy vale. Watch for another slide cascade and plunge pool at 0.6 mile.

Come to a trail intersection at 0.7 mile. Here, the Fiery Gizzard Trail heads left across a bridge over Little Fiery Gizzard Creek, while the Grundy Forest Day Loop keeps straight. For now, cross the bridge toward Sycamore Falls on the Fiery Gizzard Trail. Soon find the confluence of Big Fiery Gizzard Creek and Little Fiery Gizzard Creek. The combined water of the two streams slices a narrow slit of lathering whitewater through a sandstone cleft known as the Black Canyon.

Overhead, mountain laurel, beech, holly, and tulip trees thicken the gorge. Moss grows on anything that doesn't move. The trail is forced to climb above a creekside bluff, then navigates a boulder jumble to reach Chimney Rocks, a series of columnar sandstone monoliths 25–60 feet high. They rise to the right of the trail, where Little Fiery Gizzard Creek is working around a sharp bend. Soon come to a trail junction at 1.2 miles. Take the blue-blazed spur toward Sycamore Falls. The Fiery Gizzard Trail leaves left. Arrive at Sycamore Falls at 1.3 miles. The white curtain of water spills 15 feet from a stony brim. Add some repose time in this natural glen.

Backtrack 0.6 mile from Sycamore Falls to the Grundy Forest Day Loop. Now, head left, rising above the confluence of Little and Big Fiery Gizzard Creeks. Trace Big Fiery Gizzard Creek upstream. At 2.1 miles reach Hanes Hole Falls. The trail brings you above the gush, availing an interesting perspective as the waterfall loudly tumbles over a smooth stone lip.

Turn away from the creek at 2.2 miles, ascending in pine-hickory-oak woods. At 2.5 miles meet the spur trail leading left to the historic CCC campsite.

In the 1930s a camp of young men was located here, working on this very trail. Today, it's a backcountry campsite. Campers are required to preregister online.

Continue east, then north, then east again in the woodland, passing a small dug pond and then bridging an intermittent streamlet at 2.7 miles. The easy walking continues. Bridge Schoolhouse Branch at 2.9 miles. A hard-to-see waterfall dives 20 feet over the plateau rim here. Step across open rock slabs bordered by lichens before emerging near the trailhead picnic shelter at 3 miles, completing the loop.

Nearby Attractions

The South Cumberland State Park Visitor Center is 2.2 miles west on US 41 from the turn for Grundy State Forest. It offers maps, displays, and information about other hiking destinations on the Cumberland Plateau.

Directions

From Chattanooga, take I-24 west to Exit 135 near Monteagle. Join US 41 Alt south toward Tracy City for 0.5 mile to join US 41 south. Stay with US 41 south toward Tracy City. Hit your odometer as you pass the South Cumberland State Park Visitor Center on your left (or better yet stop and get information). Drive 2.2 miles beyond the visitor center to turn right on 3rd Street. Follow 3rd Street 0.4 mile, then turn right on Marion Street. Follow Marion Street, which then turns into Fairground Street, 0.1 mile, then turn right on Fiery Gizzard Road to dead-end at the trailhead, passing the overflow parking area. The trailhead offers restrooms, picnic tables, and a shelter.

16   Greeter Falls

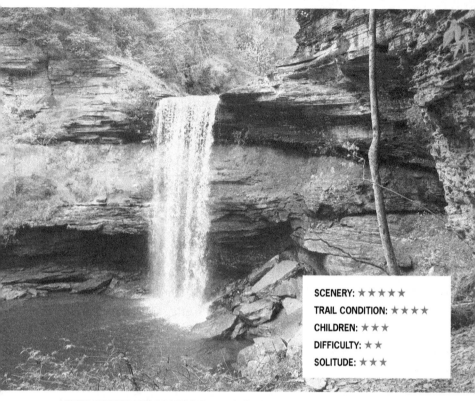

SCENERY: ★ ★ ★ ★ ★
TRAIL CONDITION: ★ ★ ★ ★
CHILDREN: ★ ★ ★
DIFFICULTY: ★ ★
SOLITUDE: ★ ★ ★

LOWER GREETER FALLS DIVES INTO AN AMPHITHEATER OF ROCK.

GPS TRAILHEAD COORDINATES: N35° 26.306' W85° 41.866'

DISTANCE & CONFIGURATION: 2.1-mile loop with spur

HIKING TIME: 1.4 hours

HIGHLIGHTS: Four waterfalls, old homesite, swimming hole

ELEVATION: 1,830' at trailhead, 1,610' at low point

ACCESS: No fees, permits, or passes required

MAPS: *South Cumberland State Park—Savage Gulf*; USGS *Altamont*

FACILITIES: None

WHEELCHAIR ACCESS: None

CONTACTS: South Cumberland State Park, 931-924-2980, tnstateparks.com/parks/south-cumberland

Overview

This hike is more than a walk to one waterfall. You will visit four cataracts, the homesite of the Greeter family, and an old-fashioned swimming hole, all on a 2-mile circuit! First, drop to the Blue Hole, a rock-rimmed pool on Firescald Creek. Backtrack to the main loop, stopping by the Greeter homesite. Begin your waterfall tour, first reaching Upper Boardtree Falls, then Lower Boardtree Falls. Next comes Lower Greeter Falls, a personal favorite of mine, then Upper Greeter Falls, a wide cascade.

Route Details

Pick up the wide Greeter Falls Loop Trail, passing around a pole gate, walking among pines and oaks. Soon come to the Blue Hole Trail. Leave right on this singletrack path, on a gentle downgrade. Hemlocks, maples, and holly add biodiversity to the pines and oaks. Ahead, step over a shallow streambed via a boardwalk, then walk atop open rock slabs. The path steepens as it passes a small rock shelter to the left of the trail and then meets Firescald Creek at 0.5 mile. The creek will run most of the year, but it can nearly dry up in late summer and fall. However, the Blue Hole will always be full. Boulders line the creek, and you have to walk downstream a bit before reaching the natural swimming pool. Rock bluffs, evergreens, and a sunning beach stand on the far side of the Blue Hole.

Backtrack to the Greeter Falls Loop Trail, turning right to shortly meet the spur trail leading left to the Greeter homesite. The Greeter family resided here in the late 1800s and early 1900s, giving their name to the nearby falls. A clearing surrounds the cut-stone foundation, and steps lead to what was a basement. The large, circular, stone-lined well is covered. Imagine the locale being much more open during the Greeters' day, with fields and farm animals, and likely a garden too. Now, the woods have crept up, and only maintenance by park personnel keeps the homesite from being overwhelmed by the inexorable vegetation of the Cumberland Plateau.

At 1.1 miles reach the actual loop portion of the hike. Stay left here, still on an old roadbed. At 1.3 miles come to another trail junction. Here, the Greeter Trail leaves left to Alum Gap and the Stone Door Ranger Station of Savage Gulf State Natural Area. Your hike leaves right, descending to Boardtree Branch,

Greeter Falls

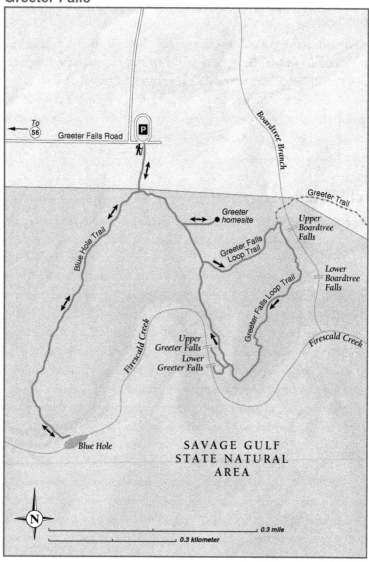

then to Upper Boardtree Falls. A spur leads left to the falls. Reach the water in midcascade. Above you, Upper Boardtree Falls spills over a widening rock face. It gathers briefly in a pool, then pours over a lip in a sheer drop below. This lip protrudes quite a bit, and a rock house (natural rock shelter) sits beneath the second part of the fall. Continue down Boardtree Branch among the rock houses and bluffs. Lower Boardtree Falls roars to your left, but the cascade is not visible from the trail. It's a tough trek to see this fall.

At 1.6 miles reach the intersection with the two Greeter Falls. Here, spurs head to Upper Greeter Falls and Lower Greeter Falls. Hike to Upper Greeter Falls first; it's a short downhill walk. This uppermost cataract pours 20 feet over a stone bluff, landing in a pool with a gigantic boulder in it. Imagine the splash made by that boulder as it landed in Firescald Creek! This is a warm-up for the superlative lower falls. To reach Lower Greeter Falls you descend a seemingly out-of-place metal staircase, the circular silver stairway that takes you down a vertical bluff to solid ground below. Follow more stairs and steps to the base of Lower Greeter Falls. Before you, a stone-walled amphitheater encircles a huge pool into which Lower Greeter Falls pours 50 feet, landing in a froth of white, then reverberates in expanding waves. Stilled massive boulders and assorted sycamores and other flora complement the picture. I believe this is one of the most beautiful places on the Cumberland Plateau.

Resume the loop, heading uphill to a break in a bluffline. Rock houses overhang the trail. The carving of Firescald Creek has left many a geological wonder in its wake. Eventually climb onto less rocky woods above the gorge. Complete the loop portion of the hike at 2 miles. From here it is a simple back-track to the trailhead.

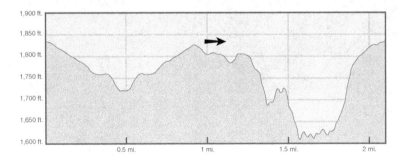

Nearby Attractions

If the hike isn't long enough, combine this hike with trails at the nearby Stone Door entrance of Savage Gulf State Natural Area.

Directions

From Exit 127 on I-24 near Pelham, take TN 50 east to Altamont. From Altamont, join TN 56 north and follow it 1.2 miles to Greeter Falls Road. Turn right on Greeter Falls Road and follow it 0.6 mile to the trailhead parking, on your left.

Alternate directions: From Whitwell, take TN 108 north 22 miles to intersect TN 56. Turn right on TN 56 north and follow it to Altamont and intersect TN 50. From this intersection, stay with TN 56 north and follow it 1.2 miles to Greeter Falls Road. Turn right on Greeter Falls Road and follow it 0.6 mile to the trailhead parking, on your left.

THIS SILVER STAIRWAY LEADS DOWN TO LOWER GREETER FALLS.

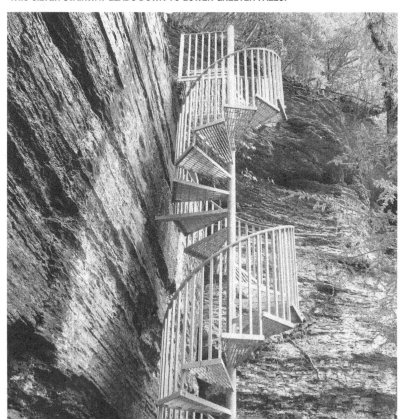

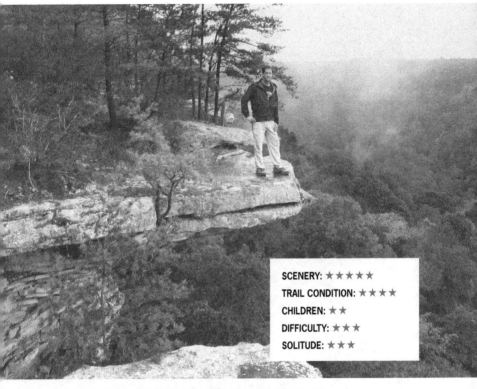

SCENERY: ★ ★ ★ ★ ★
TRAIL CONDITION: ★ ★ ★ ★
CHILDREN: ★ ★
DIFFICULTY: ★ ★ ★
SOLITUDE: ★ ★ ★

THE AUTHOR STANDS ATOP AN OUTCROP AT THE GREAT STONE DOOR.

GPS TRAILHEAD COORDINATES: N35° 26.799' W85° 39.343'

DISTANCE & CONFIGURATION: 7-mile loop with short miniloop

HIKING TIME: 4 hours

HIGHLIGHTS: Great Stone Door, multiple overlooks, moonshine still site, waterfall

ELEVATION: 1,800' at trailhead, 1,705' at low point

ACCESS: No fees, permits, or passes required

MAPS: *South Cumberland Recreation Area;* USGS *Altamont*

FACILITIES: Water, picnic area, walk-in tent camping at trailhead

WHEELCHAIR ACCESS: On first part of hike

CONTACTS: South Cumberland State Park–Savage Gulf, 931-924-2980, tnstateparks.com/parks
/south-cumberland

Stone Door Circuit

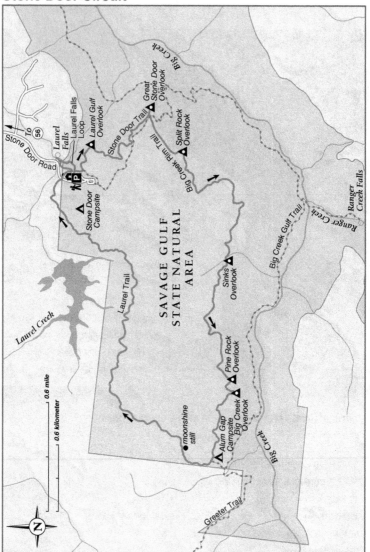

Overview

This loop first reaches one of Tennessee's finest panoramas, the Great Stone Door Overlook. A colossal sandstone slab presents multiple views of Savage Gulf State Natural Area, with its multiple gorges, Laurel Creek Gulf, Big Creek

Gulf, Collins Gulf, and Savage Gulf. More vistas await along the Big Creek Rim. Turn away from the bluffs, passing an old moonshine still site. Roll through oak stands, then make one last miniloop to view Laurel Falls and an old gristmill site.

Route Details

This is a good first longer hike. It has no major elevation changes yet delivers highlights aplenty. And the highlights start quickly. Leave the Stone Door parking area on a hard surface path, passing the Stone Door Ranger Station. Stay with the asphalt Stone Door Trail heading right, as the short Laurel Falls Loop leads left. You'll tackle that at hike's end. White oaks preside over evergreens of pine, holly, and hemlock. Dogwoods brighten spring woods, and maples add red in fall. Laurel Gulf widens to your left, and you reach the Laurel Gulf Overlook after a quarter mile. Enriching vistas open to the southeast. The all-access asphalt ends here. Resume on a wide, well-used natural-surface trail. Wooden footbridges span normally dry streambeds at 0.5 mile, 0.6 mile, and 0.7 mile.

Rise a bit, coming to a trail junction at 0.9 mile. The Big Creek Rim Trail heads right. That is your loop route, but first explore the area. The Big Creek Gulf Trail leads right and down through the Great Stone Door. View the hundreds of stone steps leading through the Great Stone Door, a crack 10 feet wide and 100 feet deep leading into Big Creek Gulf. It has been used for centuries, first by American Indians and later by settlers, to access the gulfs below. Imagine all those who have walked through the Great Stone Door before us. The Great Stone Door Overlook is dead ahead. Walk out and soak in the several panoramas from the massive sandstone slab dotted with stunted conifers. Landscapes

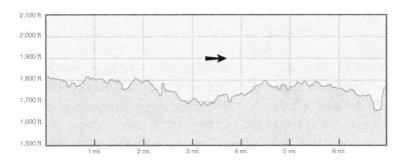

open into the heart of the natural area. Big Creek Gulf lies below and opens into a huge flat where Savage Creek, Big Creek, and the Collins River meet, making an even deeper gorge as the Collins River heads north from the Cumberland Plateau. The sheer bluffs of Big Creek Gulf are easily visible. You will shortly be walking above them.

Take the Big Creek Rim Trail southwesterly along the north rim of Big Creek Gulf, shaded by mountain laurel, pines, and oaks. Blueberry bushes grow along the brow. If you are lucky enough to catch the mountain laurel in bloom in early May, then you will be in for a treat. If hiking then, simply call the ranger station and ask about the laurel blooms. At 1.2 miles come to Split Rock Overlook, the first of many vistas along this trail. Begin a pattern of dipping into tributaries—most often dry—and then turning out to the rim. When hiking through these hickory-pine-oak forests, it is hard to imagine a drop hundreds of feet deep is nearby.

Reach the Sinks Overlook at 2.4 miles. This refers to the Big Creek Sink below, into which Big Creek flows underground most of the year. To the west, Big Creek Gulf is closing in. Come to Pine Rock Overlook at 3.3 miles, with a rewarding vista down the gulf. Also check out the nearby overhanging bluffs. You will likely hear Big Creek flowing below because you are now upstream of the sink. At 3.5 miles meet Big Creek Overlook. Big Creek Rim Trail reaches the Alum Gap backcountry campsite at 3.9 miles. Individual campsites are scattered in the surrounding woods. Just ahead is a major trail junction. Here, Big Creek Gulf Trail heads left for Big Creek. A ranger access road leads right. Greeter Trail comes in just a short distance down the Big Creek Gulf Trail, and Laurel Trail keeps straight.

Join the singletrack Laurel Trail, turning north in pine-oak woodland. Shortly bridge a wetland on a boardwalk. At 4.2 miles come to the signed remains of a moonshining operation. Two cooking areas stand side by side. At 4.9 miles the loop nears a field and the park boundary. Begin crossing numerous wetlands on boardwalks between low hills. Enjoy an extended stroll in upland forest. Walk under a power line, then cross Stone Door Road at 6.6 miles. Come alongside Laurel Gulf, then rise a bit. You pass very near the ranger station, but don't end the hike yet. Instead, turn left on the Laurel Falls Loop. Descend to a short spur to an old gristmill site. Here, you can see remains of the mill dam.

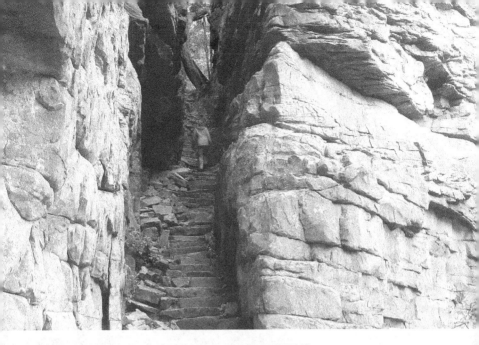

A HIKER ASCENDS THE STONE STEPS OF THE GREAT STONE DOOR.

Turn downstream and find Laurel Falls. It dives off a stone lip into a semicircular amphitheater with a huge rock house (natural rock shelter). Don't even try to reach the base of the falls in this rugged terrain. Pass a wooden observation platform before making a final short climb to the ranger station and trailhead.

Nearby Attractions

The Stone Door area offers other trails exploring Savage Gulf, as well as opportunities for backpacking.

Directions

From Exit 127 on I-24 near Pelham, take TN 50 east to Altamont. From Altamont, join TN 56 north and follow it 5.5 miles to Stone Door Road. Turn right on Stone Door Road and follow it 1 mile to enter Savage Gulf, then dead-end at the Stone Door Trailhead after 0.4 more mile.

Alternate directions: From Whitwell, take TN 108 north 22 miles to intersect TN 56. Turn right on TN 56 north and follow it to Altamont and intersect TN 50. From this intersection, follow the above directions.

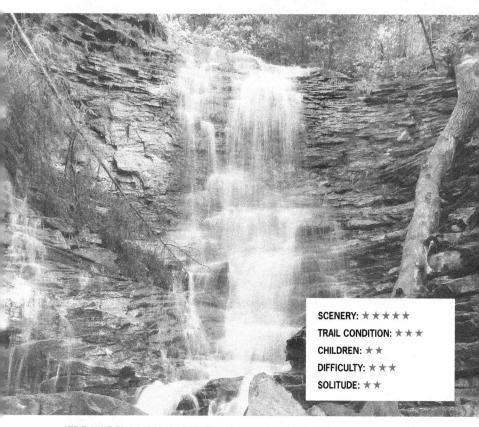

SCENERY: ★ ★ ★ ★ ★
TRAIL CONDITION: ★ ★ ★
CHILDREN: ★ ★
DIFFICULTY: ★ ★ ★
SOLITUDE: ★ ★

STRIP MINE FALLS IS MUCH PRETTIER THAN ITS NAME IMPLIES.

GPS TRAILHEAD COORDINATES: N35° 14.255' W85° 14.072'

DISTANCE & CONFIGURATION: 4.6-mile out-and-back

HIKING TIME: 3 hours

HIGHLIGHTS: Mountain creek, waterfalls, mining remains, view

ELEVATION: 790' at trailhead, 1,550' at high point

ACCESS: No fees, permits, or passes required

MAPS: Cumberland Trail—Three Gorges: North Chickamauga; USGS Daisy, Soddy, Fairmount

FACILITIES: None

WHEELCHAIR ACCESS: None

CONTACTS: Justin P. Wilson Cumberland Trail State Park, 423-566-2229, cumberlandtrail.org

Overview

This well-loved hike traces the Cumberland Trail into a deep gorge carved by North Chickamauga Creek. Enter the mouth of the gorge, hiking alongside the scrappy boulder-choked watercourse. Come to a former mine, including an old shaft and tipple remains. Strip Mine Falls tumbles over the rim in the mine vicinity. Traverse a geologically fascinating cliffline, then climb to the rim on wooden stairs. Reach a wide rock slab and gorge view. Your backtrack will yield more unseen rewards.

Route Details

Note: This is one of the most heavily used parts of the Cumberland Trail and can be quite busy on nice weekends. Consider visiting during off times. Swimmers also ply North Chickamauga Creek in summer. Law enforcement strictly enforces a no-alcohol policy to help prevent accidents in the gorge. This area was first protected as a pocket wilderness, established by Bowater Paper Company. It is now part of Cumberland Trail State Park and part of Tennessee's master path traversing the state from Signal Point in our area north to Cumberland Gap at the Kentucky–Tennessee state line.

The hike starts on a wide doubletrack path at the north end of the large parking area. The white-blazed Cumberland Trail passes picnic tables situated beside North Chickamauga Creek, where vast, clear pools slow amid massive boulders, divided by white rapids. Open rock slabs attract sunbathers. Beyond the stream, sheer walls and rock houses (natural rock shelters) rise from Chickamauga Gulch, as the valley is formally named on USGS topographic maps.

At 0.1 mile the Hogskin Branch Loop leaves right. You can use it for an alternate return route. For now, stay straight with the Cumberland Trail, heading deeper into the gulf. At 0.4 mile the old auto road you have been following leaves left to ford North Chickamauga Creek. Our route leaves right and uphill, now a singletrack path.

Turn away from the stream to ascend through rich hardwoods that color the gorge in fall. Come to Hogskin Branch. At normal flows, the tributary is more rock than water, but when flowing strong, as it can in winter and spring, Hogskin Branch will be one continuous cascade. Beyond the branch, the Cumberland Trail ascends sharply, parallel to the stream. At 0.8 mile level off at an old mine

Chickamauga Gulch Hike

access road. Here, the other end of the Hogskin Branch Loop leaves right back toward the trailhead. This hike turns left, tracing the mine access road on a moderate ascent. Reach a conspicuous overhanging rock house at 0.9 mile.

In winter you will enjoy views of the rock-rimmed gorge while passing more impressive bluffs. Reach the concrete abutments of an old coal tipple at 1.3 miles. Imagine this area bustling as an active coal mine. Curve into a stream-bed. Here a spur leads right to Strip Mine Falls. After rains, the falls drops in two curtains over a rock rim, then tumbles in stages across the trail and down below. Look for huge and well-used rock houses on the bluff just past Strip Mine Falls. At 1.4 miles look for a mineshaft to the right of the trail. It isn't barred—resist the temptation to enter. Chickamauga Gulch was both strip-mined and deep-mined. Keep hiking along the base of a cliffline, replete with overhangs, bluffs, and other geological curiosities. Don't forget to glance back down the gulch where you can gaze into the Tennessee Valley beyond the gulch mouth.

The uneven terrain, fallen boulders, and mountain slope make the going slow. Pass directly under a rock house with a horizontal roof at 2.2 miles. Here, the Cumberland Trail turns right, using stairs and wooden walkways to surmount the rim of the gorge.

After topping out, soon reach Rogers Creek Overlook. A short spur leads to a large terraced stone expanse. Rogers Creek, the view's namesake, cuts a chasm directly across the viewpoint, as does Boston Branch. More vistas open to the north, up the gorge. A house has been constructed across the gorge. The land on this side was donated to the state of Tennessee by Bowater in 2007, providing a constant passageway for the Cumberland Trail. On your return, consider taking the Hogskin Branch Loop, which leads across Hogskin Branch on the old mine road. Ahead, the loop drops right from the mine access road to switchback downhill back to the Cumberland Trail near Chickamauga Creek.

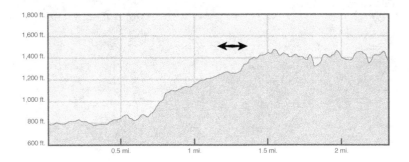

Nearby Attractions

Parcels of the Cumberland Trail extend north from here. For more options visit cumberlandtrail.org.

Directions

From the intersection of TN 153 and US 27 just north of Chattanooga, take US 27 north 2 miles to the Thrasher Pike exit. Take Thrasher Pike west 0.7 mile to Dayton Pike and a traffic light. Turn right on Dayton Pike and follow it 0.7 mile to bridge North Chickamauga Creek, then reach a traffic light and Montlake Drive. Turn left on Montlake Road (the right turn will be Industrial Park Drive) and follow it 1.1 miles to turn left into a large parking area. The Cumberland Trail starts at the far end of the parking area.

ONE OF THE MANY WET-WEATHER WATERFALLS ALONG CHICKAMAUGA GULCH

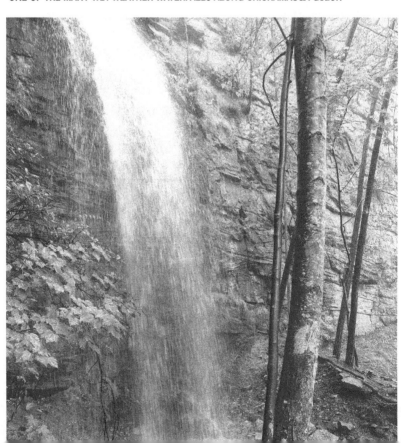

Cumberland Escarpment Hike

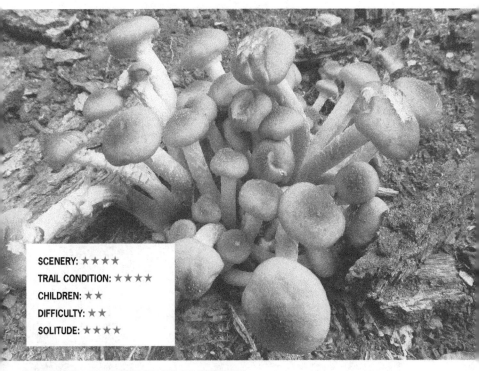

SCENERY: ★ ★ ★ ★
TRAIL CONDITION: ★ ★ ★ ★
CHILDREN: ★ ★
DIFFICULTY: ★ ★
SOLITUDE: ★ ★ ★ ★

WILD BEAUTY COMES IN PACKAGES BIG AND SMALL.

GPS TRAILHEAD COORDINATES: N35° 15.294' W85° 12.155'

DISTANCE & CONFIGURATION: 6.6-mile out-and-back

HIKING TIME: 4 hours

HIGHLIGHTS: View, American Indian rock shelters, mining history

ELEVATION: 1,650' at trailhead, 1,330' at low point

ACCESS: No fees, permits, or passes required

MAPS: *Cumberland Trail—Three Gorges: Soddy Section;* USGS *Soddy*

FACILITIES: None

WHEELCHAIR ACCESS: None

CONTACTS: Justin P. Wilson Cumberland Trail State Park, 423-566-2229, cumberlandtrail.org

Cumberland Escarpment Hike

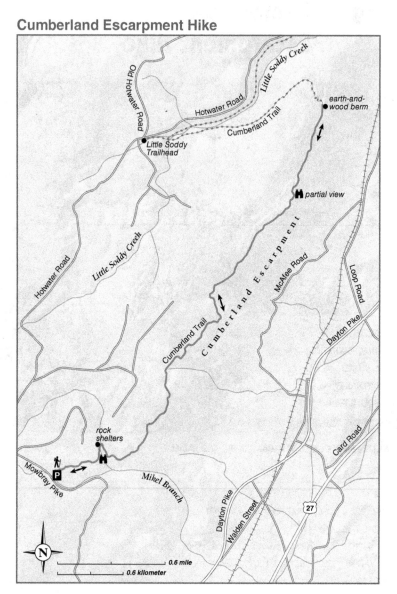

Overview

Trace the Cumberland Trail along the eastern edge of the Cumberland Escarpment above the community of Soddy-Daisy. The highlights come early. Reach a rock bluff where views open in a power line clearing. Come to Mikel Branch, where ancient and historic rock shelters border the creek. Bisect the Little Stone Door, coming to another shelter. From here, wander the wooded escarpment edge, enjoying partial views before reaching a recovering mine area near Clemmons Point.

Route Details

The main highlights are front-loaded on this hike, coming within the first half mile. But since you are up here, you may as well stretch your legs on the Cumberland Trail, Tennessee's master path. The balance of the hike travels amid eye-pleasing woodland speckled with rock gardens and ramparts characteristic of the Cumberland Plateau—and partial views of the expansive Tennessee River Valley. You will reach a long-recovered mining area from the faint past, now covered in forest, demonstrating the remarkable recuperative powers of Mother Nature. A short walk to the early highlights only is an option hikers can also consider. It is but 1 mile there and back to the view, the rock shelters, and the Little Stone Door. That would be an ideal trek for little hikers or less able adults.

Leave the Mowbray Pike Trailhead on a singletrack path, entering a xeric forest of shortleaf pine, black gum, dogwood, and red maple. Climb just a bit, then descend to step over a normally dry streambed. At 0.3 mile open onto a power line clearing. As you ramble along the edge of the Cumberland Escarpment, views open at a rock ledge. Here, the clearing reveals extensive easterly views into the Tennessee River Valley, the Sequoyah Nuclear Plant cooling towers, and beyond to the Appalachians. Although the opening is artificial, the views remain rewarding. Notice the exposed rock outcrops in other parts of the clearing.

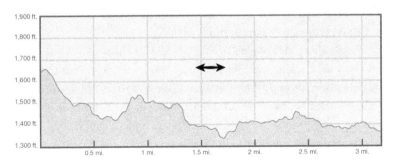

Reenter full-blown forest and shortly descend to Mikel Branch—you can hear its aquatic intonations. Explore downstream of the trail crossing. Here, you will find a pair of rock overhangs—situated on either side of Mikel Branch—that face one another. This is one of the more unusual geological wonderments of the Cumberland Plateau, dueling shelters divided by a creek. Relatively low flat roofs keep both shelters dry. Rejoin the Cumberland Trail as it turns downstream with Mikel Branch, yet well above the watercourse, which falls in cascades. At 0.4 mile the path enters a boulder garden, soon squeezing through the Little Stone Door, a slender passage between boulders. After emerging from the Little Stone Door, look left for a spur trail leading uphill a short distance to yet another rock shelter. This is the one believed to have been used by aboriginal Tennesseans.

Begin a northeasterly cruise along the escarpment of the Cumberland Plateau. Take note of the many ramparts and clifflines above. Generally the slope drops off to the right as you work around drainages heading to the valley and civilization below. Beardcane, sparkleberry, pine, and sourwood cloak the hillsides. While walking, look for unnatural land patterns, test holes, abandoned roadbeds, and other mining evidence. You may also see bits of coal washed down from above. Coal was first mined from this area beginning in 1826, but large-scale extraction started in the late 1860s with the establishment of Soddy Coal Company. At one time more than 500 men were employed, extracting coal and processing it into coke. The name *Soddy* comes from Soddy Creek. Settlers changed the Cherokee name for the stream—*Sauta*—into *Soddy,* and the name remains today.

At 1 mile pass a pair of cabin-size boulders near the trail. Imagine these boulders falling from above. At 1.2 miles cross one of many intermittent streambeds. At 1.3 miles the Cumberland Trail turns sharply but briefly downhill, only to resume its mostly level course. Watch for old coal-day relicts, now half hidden by vegetation from greenbrier to sturdy oaks.

Saddle alongside the pine-clad rocky rim of the escarpment at 1.7 miles. Ideal views always seem just out of reach between the trees, but the sounds from below drift through the vegetation. Winter views will be near constant. Wander between occasional rocks and boulders, where the trailside stonework is much appreciated. At 2.4 miles come directly below a cliffline. At 2.6 miles reach a partial view of the lowlands, Chickamauga Lake, and distant mountains.

The trail then joins a narrow artificial ridge, growing dense with trees. To your left extends a long-mined area, now completely grown over and resembling a perched narrow valley. To your right, the escarpment continues to drop off. At 2.9 miles the trail dips to an outflow of this perched valley. Continue beyond here, riding again on the artificial ridge, which becomes almost a knife edge. Drop again at 3.2 miles, crossing another outflow on an elevated earth-and-wood berm. This is a good place to turn around. From here, the Cumberland Trail ascends, then works around Clemmons Point to enter Little Soddy Creek gorge.

Nearby Attractions

Sections of the Cumberland Trail extend north from here. You can also access other mining history from the trailhead off Hotwater Road. For more options visit cumberlandtrail.org.

Directions

From Chattanooga, take US 27 north toward Soddy-Daisy. Set your odometer where TN 153 and US 27 converge. Continue north on US 27 for 4 miles to the Harrison Lane exit. Turn left (west), off US 27 to reach Dayton Pike and a traffic light. Turn right on Dayton Pike and follow it north 0.5 mile. Turn left on Mountain Road/Mowbray Pike and follow it 2.5 miles to the trailhead on your right. Watch carefully, as the trailhead will sneak up on you. If you come to Hotwater Road you have gone too far.

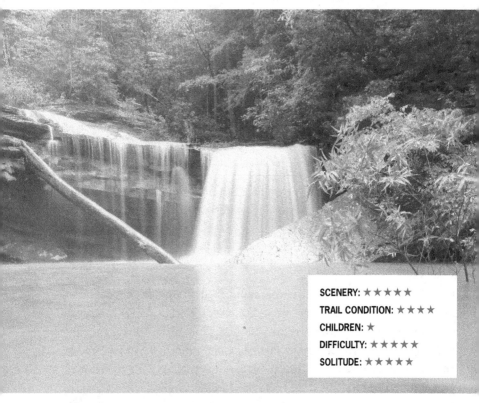

SCENERY: ★ ★ ★ ★ ★
TRAIL CONDITION: ★ ★ ★ ★
CHILDREN: ★
DIFFICULTY: ★ ★ ★ ★ ★
SOLITUDE: ★ ★ ★ ★ ★

IMODIUM FALLS GETS ITS NAME FROM THE SICK-IN-THE-STOMACH FEELING THAT DARING KAYAKERS GET BEFORE THEY PADDLE OVER THE FALLS.

GPS TRAILHEAD COORDINATES: N35° 20.752' W85° 10.505'

DISTANCE & CONFIGURATION: 9.6-mile out-and-back

HIKING TIME: 6 hours

HIGHLIGHTS: Imodium Falls, view, remote gorges, solitude, geology

ELEVATION: 1,475' at trailhead, 980' at low point

ACCESS: No fees, permits, or passes required

MAPS: *Cumberland Trail—Three Gorges: Possum Section;* USGS *Soddy*

FACILITIES: None

WHEELCHAIR ACCESS: None

CONTACTS: Justin P. Wilson Cumberland Trail State Park, 423-566-2229, cumberlandtrail.org

Overview

This remote section of the Cumberland Trail explores a craggy parcel of the Cumberland Plateau, a land where clear streams and rock overhangs cut through rich forests, where mining history adds another layer to the landscape. Hikers are challenged with a rocky trail that is rarely level. Start by tracing Blanchard Creek to bridge Big Possum Creek, then hike below a long cliffline. Soak in a vista near Perkins Point. Turn into Little Possum Creek Gorge, reaching remarkable Stack Rock. Walk along a now-wooded strip mine. Leave the mined area and reach the cleverly named Imodium Falls, a worthy destination.

Route Details

Give yourself ample time to return to the trailhead. Leave north on the Cumberland Trail from Heiss Mountain Road, immediately entering woods after you pass a trailside kiosk. The highlights start immediately. Blanchard Creek tumbles in a small waterfall to your left as you sweep beyond boulder "gates" to enter the greater Possum Creek Gorge. Cross Blanchard Creek on a bridge. The singletrack path snakes downstream past big boulders and little cascades. Bisect a closed grassy roadbed after a quarter mile.

Blanchard Creek cuts a deeper gorge of its own. At 0.6 mile come beside a cliffline. Rock ramparts rise above the path. Watch for an overhanging rock house (natural rock shelter) at 0.7 mile. Curve beneath Bare Point. Barren trees allow you to see beyond the mouth of the gorge into the Tennessee River Valley, but the point isn't as naked as you may assume. Turn into Possum Creek. Switchback downhill through evergreens on hundreds of hand-placed rock steps. Pass a small cave on a rock rampart just before reaching Big Possum Creek at 1.3 miles. Span the bouldery watercourse on a sturdy wood-and-metal bridge. Take a moment to look up and down the watercourse, cutting a scenic valley.

The Cumberland Trail climbs from the stream and briefly joins an old logging railroad grade. Watch carefully as the Cumberland Trail leaves left from the rail grade as a singletrack path, then climbs to a cliffline. At 1.5 miles come under a singular rock house known as The Amphitheater. Continue along the impressive cliffline. At 1.9 miles the Cumberland Trail switchbacks and continues ascending. Circle behind Perkins Point, finally leveling off on Hughes Ridge

Possum Creek Gorge

at 2.4 miles. This trail never stays level for long. The path descends to a short spur and a view at 2.5 miles. A stone promontory opens to a panorama beyond Possum Creek Gorge and into the Tennessee River Valley. The Southern Appalachians rise as a distant backdrop. What a view!

Leave the vista and travel downhill, on a now-predictably rocky track, breaking through a cliffline, aiming for Little Possum Creek. More stone steps and switchbacks take you farther down before turning upstream into Little Possum Creek Gorge. Little Possum Creek is making its way through exceedingly craggy and mean topography. Come to a small designated backcountry campsite at 3 miles. The camp is backed up against an embedded boulder and has room for a small party.

The Cumberland Trail fights upstream in the narrowing defile. More stony steps find a long bridge spanning Little Possum Creek at 3.1 miles. The other side of the creek is also stone-filled and disheartening for a sore-footed hiker. However, the incredible scenery inspires. Reach the stone pillar known as Stack Rock at 3.4 miles. Hikers often have their picture taken here. The Cumberland Trail switchbacks and reaches the top of the rock. Step out and grab a view of the immediate Little Possum Creek Gorge.

At 3.7 miles the Cumberland Trail passes near private land and an auto-accessible camp. Join a roadbed here and begin traveling along a 1950s strip mine cut. The area has now recovered and is forested. However, the terrain remains nonnatural in appearance. Ironically, the strip mine bench makes the hiking much easier. Trace the old coal seam until 4.4 miles, returning to unaltered forestland. The Cumberland Trail descends by switchbacks toward Little Possum Creek, winding between clifflines. You will both see and hear Imodium Falls to your left at 4.8 miles. The cataract is most easily accessible from the top, but be very careful if the water is high. You will be on the horseshoe-shaped lip of the 25-foot cascade. Depending on flow levels, the falls can reveal varied faces. Big boulders stand mute in the plunge pool below. Hikers accessing the

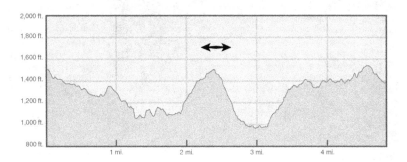

falls' base will appreciate the rock overhang over which the creek spills and the depth of the rock house (natural rock shelter) behind the falls.

Nearby Attractions

The Soddy section of the Cumberland Trail extends south from this trailhead, heading down Boardcamp Creek to Big Soddy Creek and points south.

Directions

From Chattanooga, take US 27 north to Soddy-Daisy. From the intersection of TN 111 and US 27 just north of Soddy-Daisy, take TN 111 north 4 miles to the Jones Gap Road exit. Turn right on Jones Gap Road and follow it just a short distance to turn right on Heiss Mountain Road. Follow Heiss Mountain Road 0.5 mile to reach the trailhead on your left.

FIND THESE CASCADES ON BLANCHARD CREEK.

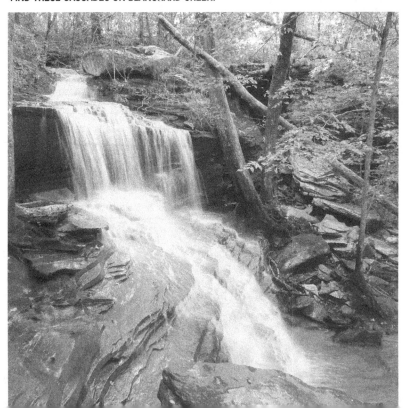

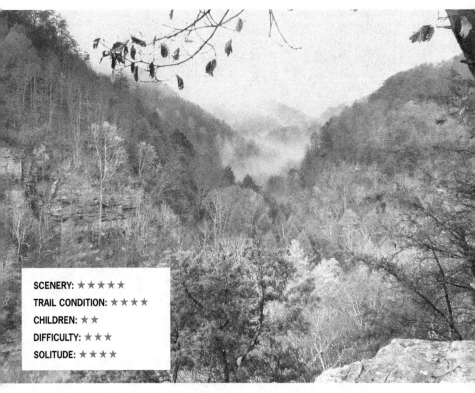

SCENERY: ★ ★ ★ ★ ★
TRAIL CONDITION: ★ ★ ★ ★
CHILDREN: ★ ★
DIFFICULTY: ★ ★ ★
SOLITUDE: ★ ★ ★ ★

ROCK CREEK GORGE ON A FOGGY FALL MORNING

GPS TRAILHEAD COORDINATES: N35° 24.580', W85° 07.850'

DISTANCE & CONFIGURATION: 4.3-mile loop

HIKING TIME: 3 hours

HIGHLIGHTS: Two vistas, gorge, solitude

ELEVATION: 1,550' at trailhead, 910' at low point

ACCESS: No fees, permits, or passes required

MAPS: *Cumberland Trail—Three Gorges: Rock Section;* USGS *Brayton*

FACILITIES: None

WHEELCHAIR ACCESS: None

CONTACTS: Justin P. Wilson Cumberland Trail State Park, 423-566-2229; tnstateparks.com

Rock Creek Gorge Loop

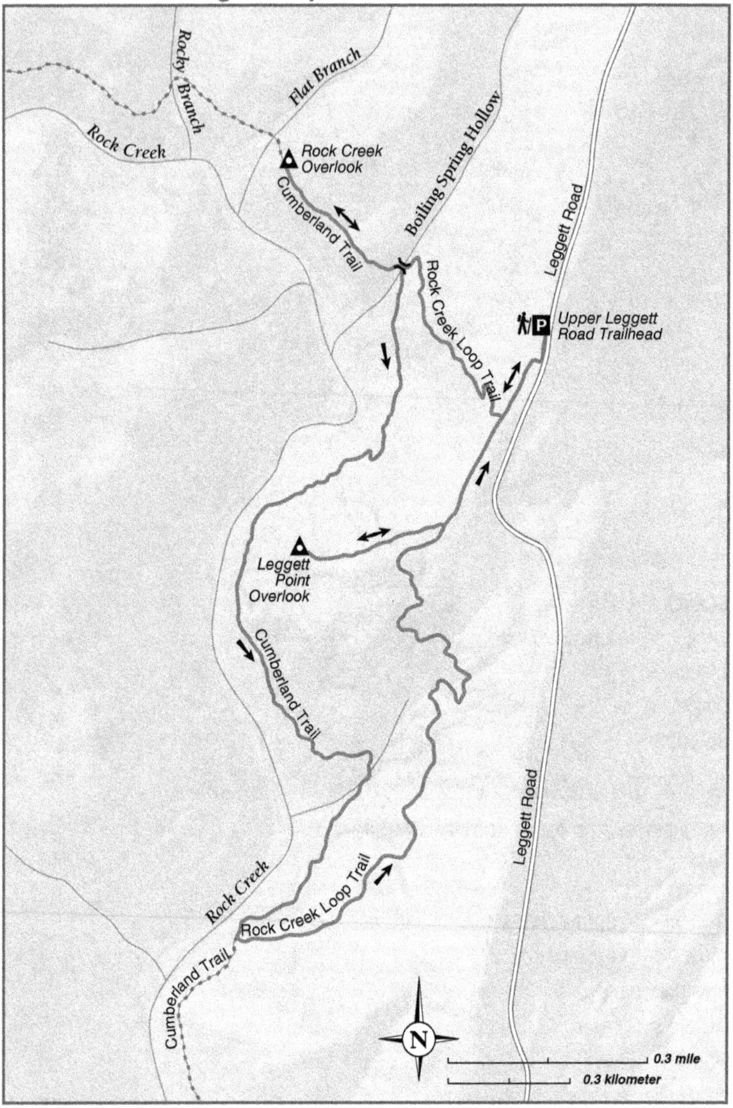

Rocky Branch
Flat Branch
Rock Creek
Rock Creek Overlook
Cumberland Trail
Boiling Spring Hollow
Leggett Road
Rock Creek Loop Trail
Upper Leggett Road Trailhead
Leggett Point Overlook
Cumberland Trail
Leggett Road
Rock Creek
Rock Creek Loop Trail
Cumberland Trail
N
0.3 mile
0.3 kilometer

Overview

This hike explores rugged Rock Creek Gorge, located in the extreme northwestern corner of Hamilton County. Start high atop the Cumberland Plateau and descend into the gorge. Detour to Rock Creek Overlook, a vista into the rock-rimmed chasm. Burrow into the lower Rock Creek Gorge on a stony path to the bottomland and creek. From there, ascend to the high country and then take a spur to Leggett Point Overlook, where you can soak in more views of Rock Creek Gorge. From the overlook it's a short distance to the trailhead.

Route Details

From the upper Leggett Road Trailhead, follow a path heading south along Leggett Road before entering the woods. Pass a trailhead signboard, and then trace an old roadbed under pines. Golden needles carpet the path as you head south. At 0.1 mile you arrive at the loop portion of the hike, Rock Creek Loop Trail. Turn right here on a blue-blazed track, aiming for Rock Creek Overlook. Descend a steep slope amid impressive rock bluffs under pines, maples, mountain laurel, and chestnut oaks. Stone steps make the irregular terrain easier on the feet, but the singletrack path is slow going. The trail work here is quite impressive.

Turn into Boiling Spring Hollow, reaching a trail intersection at 0.5 mile. Turn right here, joining the official Cumberland Trail. You will return to this point later to complete your loop, but first take a side trip out to Rock Creek Overlook. A slender, stony track heads up the Rock Creek Gorge, immediately crossing the stream that cuts Boiling Spring Hollow. Navigate an irregular, declivitous slope dotted with cedars and beard cane. When the leaves are off the trees, you can easily see the clifflines across the gorge and above you as well. However, an even better view opens up at Rock Creek Overlook, at 0.8 mile. Here, an open stone point presents views both up and down the gorge. Upstream, angled ridges alternate into the chasm. Across from you, clifflines

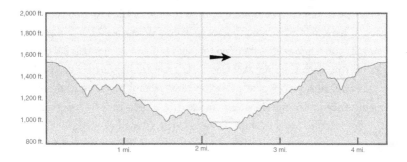

drop sharply to the gorge base, while downstream the gorge curves out of sight. But you will be there soon.

Backtrack to Boiling Spring Hollow, reaching it at 1.1 miles. Join a new section of the Cumberland Trail, heading downstream into the valley. The fluid shapes in nature are evident everywhere in this vale—the sun-following trees, the curved rocks, and the flowing stream. Bisect small drainages aiming for Rock Creek. Hemlocks, maples, and ferns become more common the lower you dip into the basin. The watercourse remains tantalizingly out of reach, though. Step over a streambed cutting a V at 2.1 miles, then turn back toward Rock Creek. Drop into bottomland at 2.2 miles.

Note the moisture-loving beech trees that populate the flat. Beech trees are among the easiest trees to identify. Their smooth gray trunks make them stand out in the forest, as carved trees will testify. Many woodland walkers simply can't resist the flat surface of the beech—it seems a tablet for a handy pocketknife. The smooth trunks contrast greatly with knobby and fissured hardwoods around them. Pick up a beech leaf from the forest floor. The sunlight-absorbing leaves are generally 2–4 inches long. Note the sharply toothed edges of the leaves. They are a dark green on top and lighter underneath. In fall, they turn a yellowish golden brown. Under ideal conditions, beech trees can reach 120 feet tall. After beech leaves fall, you will notice the buds of next year's leaves. The half-inch buds resemble a mini cigar. Come spring, these buds will unfurl to once again convert sunlight for the tree as it resumes growing.

A spur trail leads right to Rock Creek. If you want to enjoy the stream, do it now, for this hike reaches a trail junction just ahead at 2.4 miles. Here, the Cumberland Trail keeps straight and continues down the Rock Creek Gorge to the lower Leggett Road Trailhead. This hike turns left on the Rock Creek Loop Trail.

Angle upslope, northbound, still on a singletrack path. The gorge isn't as sloped here, and you wander across shallow drainages. You bridge several streams as you climb ever higher and top out on the plateau rim at 3.4 miles. At 3.5 miles you reach the spur trail leading left toward Leggett Point. Head west and downhill into young pines. Reach a rock promontory, the farthest point being distended from the ridge you are walking. A little rock-hopping takes you to the far outcrop, Leggett Point. Gaze into the ravine below. Hardwoods and pines grow where stone walls aren't. Rock Creek noisily flows, incrementally yet continually, carving the valley ever deeper.

Backtrack from the overlook, then resume the loop north. Complete the loop portion of the hike at 4.2 miles, then backtrack to the trailhead, finishing the hike.

Nearby Attractions

Parcels of the Cumberland Trail extend both north and south of this loop. For more options visit cumberlandtrail.org.

Directions

From Chattanooga, take US 27 north to Soddy-Daisy. From the intersection of TN 111 and US 27 just north of Soddy-Daisy, take US 27 north 6 miles to Leggett Road, located in the Sale Creek community. Turn left on Leggett Road and follow it 3.4 miles to the trailhead parking on your left. Do not mistakenly park in the lower Rock Creek Gorge parking area at 1.5 miles on Leggett Road.

THE CUMBERLAND TRAIL TAKES YOU THROUGH A BEAUTIFUL FOREST IN THE ROCK CREEK GORGE.

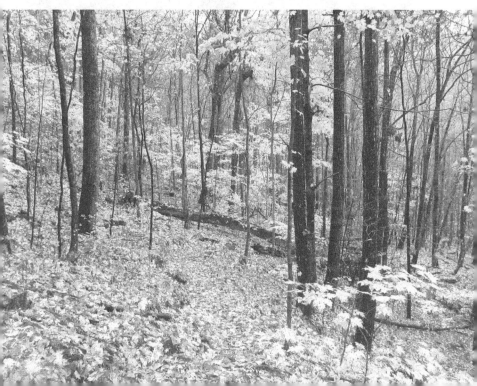

22   **Laurel Snow Waterfall and Vista Hike**

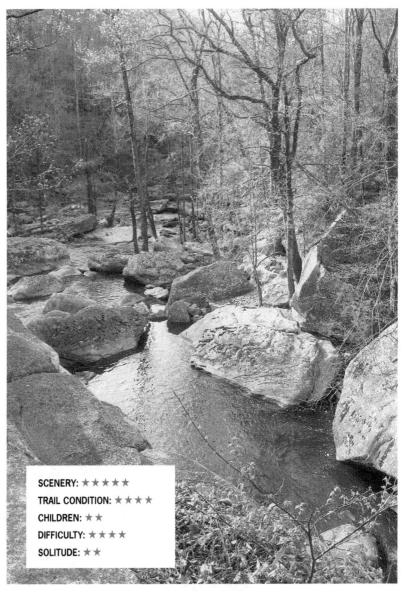

SCENERY: ★★★★★
TRAIL CONDITION: ★★★★
CHILDREN: ★★
DIFFICULTY: ★★★★
SOLITUDE: ★★

LOOKING DOWNSTREAM ON BOULDERY RICHLAND CREEK

GPS TRAILHEAD COORDINATES: N35° 31.587' W85° 01.288'

DISTANCE & CONFIGURATION: 6.2-mile out-and-back

HIKING TIME: 4 hours

HIGHLIGHTS: Richland Mine, Laurel Falls, views

ELEVATION: 920' at trailhead, 1,730' at high point

ACCESS: No fees, permits, or passes required

MAPS: Cumberland Trail—Laurel Snow Segment; USGS Morgan Springs

FACILITIES: None

WHEELCHAIR ACCESS: None

CONTACTS: Justin P. Wilson Cumberland Trail State Park, 423-566-2229, cumberlandtrail.org

Overview

This hike visits historical, aquatic, and geological highlights of Laurel Snow Wilderness, all on Tennessee's first federally designated national recreation trail. Hike up rock-walled Richland Creek valley, past the historic Richland Mine. Continuing up the gorge you will near the old Dayton Reservoir. Turn up bouldery Laurel Creek, winding up switchbacks to reach Laurel Falls, an 80-foot tumbler diving over a rock face. Climb to the gorge rim, crossing Laurel Creek to reach a pair of overlooks availing panoramas of this Cumberland Plateau treasure.

Route Details

The first part of the hike is as easy as the second half is hard. Walk north on a wide, stress-free path entering the imposing maw of the Richland Creek gorge. Richland Creek flows in rapids and pools as it slices, slips, and slides between and among gigantic boulders. Quickly bridge a tributary—Paine Creek—which falls between more big rocks. Watch for spur trails heading uphill to the lowermost part of the old Richland Mine, where a leveled flat stands complete with stonework, including a hand-crafted arch. Look for evidence of the stone mine structure visible from the main path. At 0.3 mile come near a mine opening with arched stonework at its entrance.

Despite the mining relics, the natural aspects of the Richland Creek valley overwhelm the scene. Sheer stone sentinels, towering bluffs, and rock shelters rise from the waterway. Large, flat rocks alongside Richland Creek provide

Laurel Snow Waterfall and Vista Hike

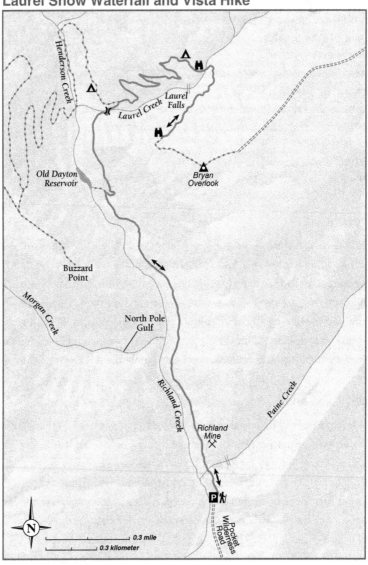

sunning spots for stream swimmers. Sweetgum, white oak, ironwood, and other hardwoods grow in less rocky spaces. At 0.5 mile an old road leads left to the confluence of Morgan Creek and Richland Creek. Naked concrete bridge abutments cross Richland Creek, absent of the span that once topped them. Morgan

Creek valley is also known as North Pole Gulf, bringing to mind the chilly circumstances that inspired this name.

The main trail penetrates deeper up Richland Creek. At 0.6 mile look for embedded railroad ties from a narrow-gauge lumber operation railroad. The exposed pipe you occasionally see remains from the old Dayton Reservoir. After 1 mile the trail narrows and slightly steepens. Look for the great walls atop the gulf rim, easily visible when the leaves have fallen. Nearby, woodland boulders stand in still repose among the trees. The stream is awash in graybacks, polished smooth by ceaseless water flow.

At 1.3 miles reach a signed intersection. Here, a spur trail to the old Dayton Reservoir keeps straight and is a popular destination for those who want an easy hike. There, you will see a concrete spillway from the old town water-storage facility. The main trail switchbacks uphill into the gorge. Pick your way through boulder fields to cross Laurel Creek on a metal bridge at 1.7 miles.

Come to another signed trail junction just ahead. Here, the Laurel Creek Trail leads right, while the trail to Snow Falls leads left. These two cataracts gave the wilderness its name—Laurel Snow. Turn right and head up Laurel Creek. Navigate up a boulder garden, tunneling by hands and feet through one boulder formation. Emerge from the brief darkness and begin a series of loping switchbacks up Laurel Creek, winding ever higher in mountainside forest. At 2.3 miles reach the short spur trail to Laurel Falls. Enjoy looking up at the chute as it tumbles from the rim of the gorge 80 feet into a boulder jumble, gathering steam, then pushing downward, eventually to meet its mother stream, Richland Creek.

Turn away from Laurel Falls, coming along the base of the gorge rim. Imposing walls rise high to your right. The trail finds a break in the rim. Here,

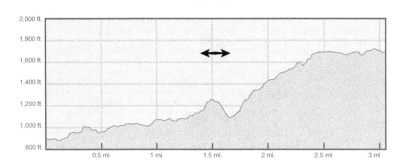

you scramble up the fissure, albeit marked and blazed. Top out in a piney flat at 2.5 miles. The trail goes but a short distance before passing a spur leading left to the designated Laurel Falls campsite.

The main trail cruises the crest of the Cumberland Plateau. The chasm of the Richland Creek gorge falls to your right. At 2.6 miles pass a marked spur trail leading right to a stone outcrop and vista. From this stony pine-framed perch, gaze westerly down the Laurel Creek gorge and beyond. At 2.7 miles the trail makes a shallow ford of Laurel Creek. In spring, you may have to shed your shoes to cross, but a crashing Laurel Falls will be your reward. The path curves southwesterly under evergreens. Open to a stone-and-pine flat and an outcrop at 3.1 miles. Walk to the edge of the precipice. In front of you, Richland Creek cuts its rift. Look across the valley at other outcrops, then back to the vista where you were at 2.6 miles. Laurel Creek Falls echoes across the valley.

Nearby Attractions

Consider timing your visit with the annual Tennessee Strawberry Festival, held in May. Check tnstrawberryfestival.com for more information.

Directions

From Chattanooga, take US 27 north to Dayton. From the intersection of US 27 and TN 30 in Dayton (traffic light #7), head north on US 27 for 1.6 miles to Walnut Grove Road (traffic light #8). Turn left on Walnut Grove Road, which turns into Back Valley Road, and follow it 1.4 miles to the signed right turn for Laurel Snow State Natural Area. The turn is across from Bethel Holiness Church. Follow gravel Pocket Wilderness Road 0.8 mile to dead-end at the trailhead.

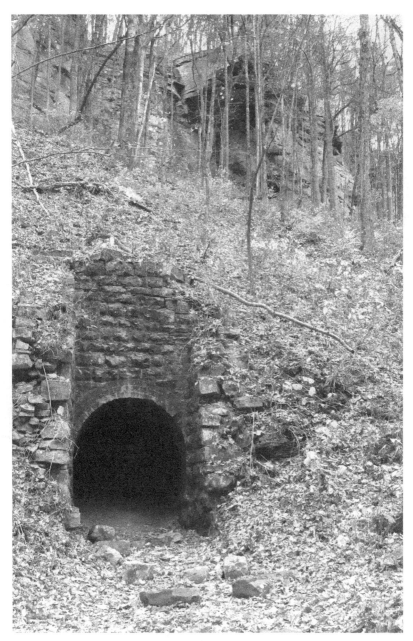

THE ARCHED OPENING OF THE RICHLAND MINE

Tennessee Appalachians (Hikes 23–29)

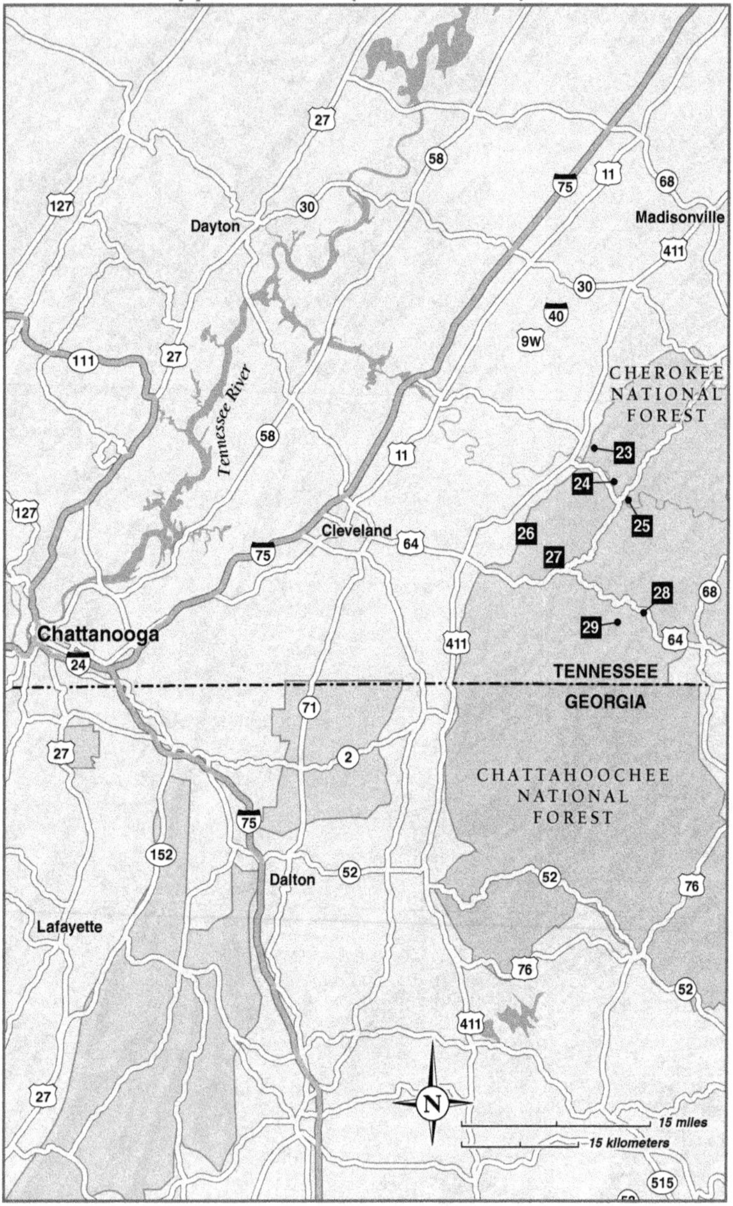
Dayton
Madisonville
Tennessee River
CHEROKEE NATIONAL FOREST
Cleveland
Chattanooga
TENNESSEE
GEORGIA
CHATTAHOOCHEE NATIONAL FOREST
Dalton
Lafayette
23
24
25
26
27
28
29
27
58
75
11
68
127
30
411
40
9W
111
64
24
71
2
152
52
76
515
15 miles
15 kilometers
N

Tennessee Appalachians

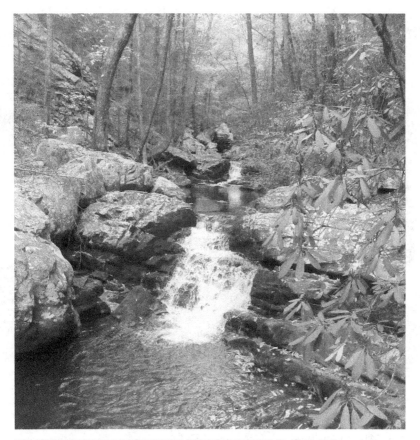

GEE CREEK DESERVES ITS WILDERNESS DESIGNATION. (HIKE 23, PAGE 136)

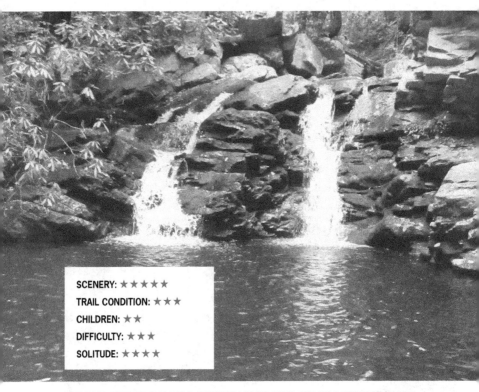

SCENERY: ★★★★★
TRAIL CONDITION: ★★★
CHILDREN: ★★
DIFFICULTY: ★★★
SOLITUDE: ★★★★

THE POOL AT TWIN FALLS IS A GREAT PLACE TO COOL OFF ON A HOT AFTERNOON.

GPS TRAILHEAD COORDINATES: N35° 14.814' W84° 32.409'

DISTANCE & CONFIGURATION: 3.8-mile out-and-back

HIKING TIME: 2.5 hours

HIGHLIGHTS: Waterfalls, rock gorge, wilderness

ELEVATION: 930' at trailhead, 1,530' at turnaround point

ACCESS: No fees, permits, or passes required

MAPS: National Geographic *Cherokee National Forest—Tellico & Ocoee Rivers;* USGS *Oswald Dome, Etowah*

FACILITIES: None

WHEELCHAIR ACCESS: None

CONTACTS: Cherokee National Forest, Ocoee Ranger District, 423-338-3300, fs.usda.gov/cherokee

Overview

Explore the incredible Gee Creek gorge. Leave the trailhead, walking on an old roadbed, and then enter the gorge. Make a seemingly instantaneous entrance into the back of beyond—a wild, high, rock- and tree-rimmed chasm. Trace a slender footpath deeper into the defile, passing an old mine, a significant waterfall, and towering stone cliffs. Multiple creek crossings on the latter half of the hike add to the excitement. The hike ends a little less than 2 miles into the gorge. Allow plenty of time for your return trip, as the trail is rocky and slow.

Route Details

The Gee Creek Wilderness, at under 2,500 acres, may be small geographically, but it is outsized in ruggedness and true wilderness feel. Established in 1975 by Congress, Gee Creek cuts a 1,000-foot gulf between Starr and Chestnut Mountains. The ruggedness of this Cherokee National Forest hidden gem isn't evident until you start into its recesses, though if you're driving north up US 411 from Chattanooga, the steepness of the V-shaped gorge is clearly visible. Prepare to be amazed at the deep pools of the small stream, the boulders, and cliffs all draped in rich lush forest.

Pass around a vehicle barrier at the trailhead, tracing a wide but rocky trail in pine-prevailing forest. Gee Creek flows well off to your right. Walk deeper into the flat. The gorge begins tightening its noose around Gee Creek. After a quarter mile the trail sidles alongside the waterway. The translucent mountain stream is born high on Starr Mountain, and its only major tributary is Poplar Springs Branch. Despite its smallish size and watershed, Gee Creek has some surprisingly deep pools that harbor feisty rainbow trout.

At 0.4 mile a user-created trail dips to a flat and a campsite. At 0.5 mile reach a wooden footbridge spanning Gee Creek. Big boulders line the streambed. You are now ascending the right bank of the watercourse. The first of many vertical walls rises from the clear-as-air stream. The hike officially enters Gee Creek Wilderness, where camping is not allowed. The path steepens underneath sycamore and hemlock in a now slender, steep chasm. Gee Creek wildly tumbles in multiple cataracts as you ascend, picking your way among boulders and trees.

Gee Creek Wilderness

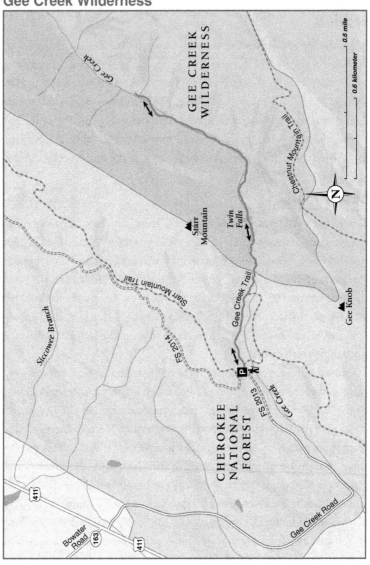

Even while peering down at the cascades, also examine the bluffs and walls of the gorge, which amplifies the booming stream.

At 0.6 mile reach a relic concrete structure and, in the creek, an old flume. These are remnants from the Tennessee Copper Company, in operation from

1825 to 1860. They weren't mining copper here, rather seeking an iron ore used in the copper smelting process. Gee Creek continues to flow through the flume, located in the streambed, except in high water when it overwhelms the flume and flows through its old bed.

Continue up the gorge. At 0.9 mile reach Twin Falls and the first stream crossing. Twin Falls tumbles in two parallel cataracts into a pool far outsizing the stream. Hikers could easily dunk themselves here. Now begins the first of eight unbridged crossings between Twin Falls and the trail's end. Even at high water or in winter you can make it here and then turn around. At normal flows, agile hikers will manage a dry-footed stream crossing. Shortly rock-hop back to the right bank. Soon reach a small but level pine glen. A sheer rock wall rises to your right and Gee Creek flows to your left. This is a superlatively scenic spot.

The path cuts deeper into the boulder-strewn chasm. At 1.2 miles clamber over a rock jutting into the waterway. Make a pair of quick stream crossings, then open into a flat on the right bank. Watch for a huge tulip tree here. The small flat closes and the path crosses left at 1.3 miles. The gorge curves northeast, now in a cooler environment with black birch and scads of rhododendron. At 1.4 miles look up the far wall of the gorge for a tributary stream dropping in a sheet flow cascade.

The main gorge is now but a slender slit, the eastern version of a slot canyon. Cross to the right bank at 1.5 miles, hiking well above the creek. Cross to the left bank at 1.7 miles. Pass serrated rock walls rising on your right. At 1.8 miles make your final crossing. You are again on the right bank. Enter a flat and here, at 1.9 miles, the trail dead-ends. A faint user-created path continues, but I recommend turning around in this wild slice of East Tennessee.

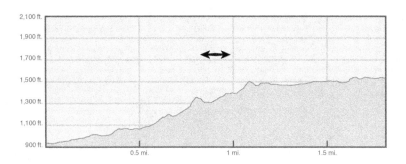

Nearby Attractions

Hiwassee/Ocoee State Scenic River Park, operated by the state of Tennessee, is located nearby. It offers attractive campsites in the flats near the Hiwassee River. Combine your hike into the Gee Creek Wilderness with a paddling or tubing trip on the river, and also camp out all in the same locale. For more information, visit tnstateparks.com.

Directions

From Exit 36 on I-75 northeast of downtown Chattanooga, take TN 163 east 15 miles to US 411 near Delano. Once at US 411, turn right (south) and go just a few feet to then turn left on Gee Creek Road. Follow Gee Creek Road over railroad tracks and stay right, continuing with Gee Creek Road as it turns back north and turns into Forest Service Road 2013. Travel a total of 2.2 miles from US 411 to reach the signed trailhead, just before a left curve.

24 Benton MacKaye Trail on the Hiwassee River

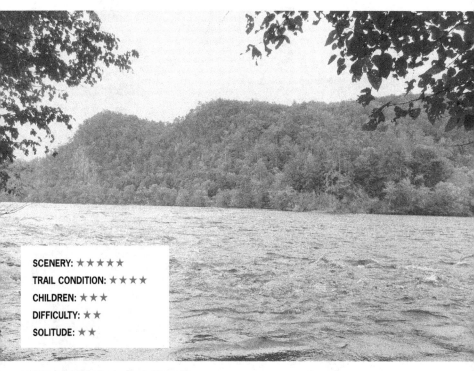

SCENERY: ★ ★ ★ ★ ★
TRAIL CONDITION: ★ ★ ★ ★
CHILDREN: ★ ★ ★
DIFFICULTY: ★ ★
SOLITUDE: ★ ★

THE WILD AND SCENIC HIWASSEE RIVER

GPS TRAILHEAD COORDINATES: N35° 11.364' W84° 29.431'

DISTANCE & CONFIGURATION: 6-mile out-and-back

HIKING TIME: 3.2 hours

HIGHLIGHTS: Tennessee Wild and Scenic River views, level track, wildflowers

ELEVATION: 760' at trailhead, 880' at high point

ACCESS: No fees, permits, or passes required

MAPS: National Geographic *Cherokee National Forest—Tellico & Ocoee Rivers*; USGS *McFarland*

FACILITIES: Restroom, picnic tables at trail's end

WHEELCHAIR ACCESS: None

CONTACTS: Cherokee National Forest, Ocoee Ranger District, 423-338-3300, fs.usda.gov/cherokee; bmta.org

Benton MacKaye Trail on the Hiwassee River

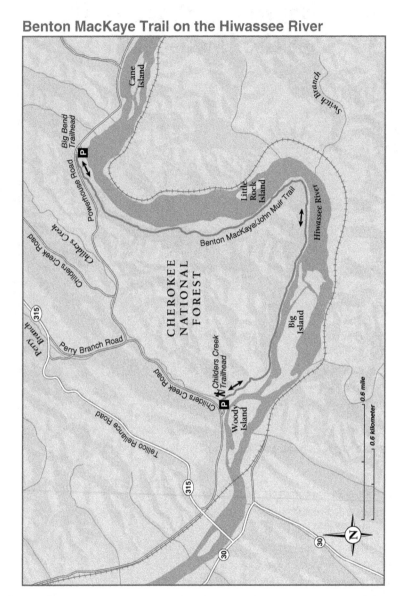

Overview

Take a relatively easy hike along the beautiful banks of the wild and scenic Hiwassee River. Head upstream from the Childers Creek Trailhead, skirting riverside woods bordered by the river on one side and rocky protuberances on the other. Cruise past islands, bluffs, and shoals as the Hiwassee makes a big bend. Look for paddlers and anglers in the river during the warm season. The hike ends at Big Bend Trailhead, availing an alternate hiker access.

Route Details

This hike traverses a stretch of the Benton MacKaye Trail (BMT), a long-distance path winding through the Southern Appalachians from Springer Mountain in North Georgia to the eastern end of the Great Smoky Mountains at Davenport Gap, providing an alternate path to the Appalachian Trail. This section of the BMT overlays the preexisting John Muir Trail. Names aside, the path provides a dry-footed way to view one of the Volunteer State's prettiest rivers, the Hiwassee. In addition, the low elevation makes for an ideal wintertime or cool-weather hike, when higher areas of the Cherokee National Forest may be excessively cold.

Leave the Childers Creek Trailhead, joining the Benton MacKaye/John Muir Trail after crossing a wooden footbridge over crystalline Childers Creek. A large flat, partly wooded in walnut trees and brush, divides you from the Hiwassee River. A steep piney hillside rises to your left. Buckeye, sweetgum, and maple shade the mostly level track, which presents easy and pleasant walking. After a quarter mile a projecting rock bluff pushes the trail alongside the banks of the Hiwassee River. Note the islands dividing the river, the largest of which is Big Island. You will see paddlers plying the Class I–III rapids when upstream Apalachia Dam (located near the Tennessee–North Carolina border) is generating power; when it's not generating, anglers may be wade fishing.

Watch for more outcrops and cliffs rising to your left. Ironwood, also known as hornbeam, rises fast along the river's edge, along with sycamore,

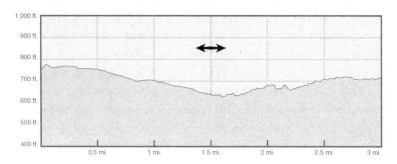

143

beech, and holly trees. A preponderance of yuccas lines the trail. You are hiking easterly. The trail stays close to the river. When islands are not present, the Hiwassee extends upwards of 200 yards across. At 1.1 miles a rock outcrop extends toward the Hiwassee, allowing views toward submerged ledges over which this mountain water spills. Ahead, the trail is squeezed again by bluffs to the left and the river to the right.

At 1.4 miles the trail bends sharply left (northwest). The exposure changes the vegetation to moister plants—doghobble, ferns, rhododendron, and some remaining hemlocks. The trail begins a few small undulations as it works over boulders and riverside hillocks. More islands appear, and you can see the CSX Railroad trudging through the gorge. At 1.7 miles come alongside an overhanging bluff and rock house (natural rock shelter). A handrail and stone steps take you back to the river's edge, where cool river breezes make a summer's day hike nigh well tolerable. Landward rock bluffs continue to amaze. At 1.8 miles the path drifts back from the river in a pawpaw-laden flat, a riverside wetland. Return to the river's edge at 2.2 miles. To your right is a campsite and paddler lunch spot below a series of watery ledges. The BMT picks up an old roadbed, and from here on out the hiking is a breeze. Work around a few more flats, then reach the Big Bend Trailhead at 3 miles. A backtrack to Childers Creek Trailhead is your best bet.

A one-way hike shuttle can be made by continuing past Childers Creek Trailhead on Childers Creek Road, then turning right, still with Childers Creek Road, then turning at the next right on Powerhouse Road to soon reach Big Bend Trailhead.

The Benton MacKaye Trail, completed in 2005, is 290 miles long. The trail is named for the man who came up with the idea for the Appalachian Trail. The footpath travels not only Tennessee, but also Georgia and North Carolina. Far fewer people have hiked the entire BMT than the Appalachian Trail, despite its much shorter length, because it's less known, less "glamorous," and seemingly easier. But mile for mile, the BMT is more challenging than the AT, due to steeper ups and downs, fewer resupply locations, and its lack of hiker hostels. No reliable statistics have been compiled on the number of BMT thru-hikers. The section in Tennessee's Cherokee National Forest is superlatively scenic as it passes through five federally designated wildernesses amid a number of rivers and mountains beyond the Hiwassee. For more information about the BMT, visit bmta.org.

Nearby Attractions

You can canoe, tube, or raft the Hiwassee with outfitters located in nearby Reliance. Anglers can vie for trout among the rapids, especially when the upstream dam is not generating power.

Directions

From Exit 36 on I-75 northeast of downtown Chattanooga, take TN 163 east 15 miles to US 411 near Delano. Once at US 411, turn right and drive 1.9 miles to TN 30, on the south side of the Hiwassee River. Turn left (east) on TN 30 and follow it 5.7 miles to the community of Reliance and TN 315. Turn left on TN 315, bridge the Hiwassee River, then turn right on Childers Creek Road and follow it 0.5 mile to the trailhead on your right.

BIRDS LOVE THE FRUIT OF THIS PLANT, COMMONLY KNOWN AS HEARTS-A-BUSTIN'.

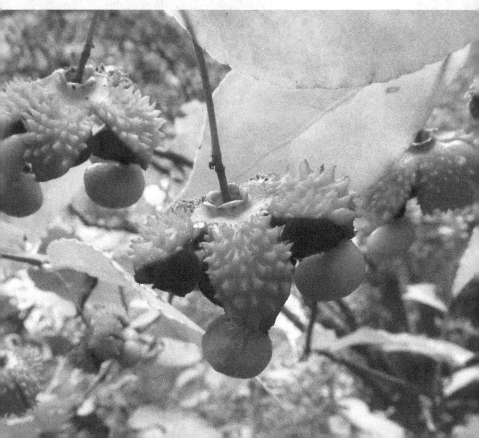

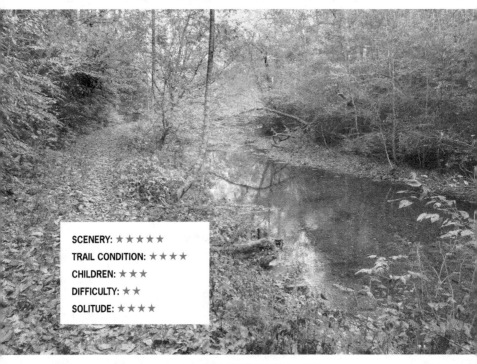

SCENERY: ★ ★ ★ ★ ★
TRAIL CONDITION: ★ ★ ★ ★
CHILDREN: ★ ★ ★
DIFFICULTY: ★ ★
SOLITUDE: ★ ★ ★ ★

BIG LOST CREEK IS A SCENIC SOUTHERN APPALACHIAN STREAM.

GPS TRAILHEAD COORDINATES: N35° 09.702' W84° 28.132'

DISTANCE & CONFIGURATION: 5.6-mile out-and-back

HIKING TIME: 2.3 hours

HIGHLIGHTS: Mountain stream, cascades

ELEVATION: 1,060' at trailhead, 773' at low point

ACCESS: No fees, permits, or passes required

MAPS: National Geographic *Cherokee National Forest—Tellico & Ocoee Rivers*; USGS *McFarland*

FACILITIES: Campground, restrooms nearby

WHEELCHAIR ACCESS: None

CONTACTS: Cherokee National Forest, Ocoee Ranger District, 423-338-3300, fs.usda.gov/cherokee; bmta.org

Overview

This adventure traverses a portion of the long-distance Benton MacKaye Trail (BMT) along beautiful Big Lost Creek, a tributary of the Hiwassee River in the Cherokee National Forest. Start your hike near Lost Creek Campground. Head downstream as the clear stream, displaying everywhere-you-look beauty, bends past former homesteads before cutting into steeper terrain where the stream cascades among boulders before calming down. Turn around when the trail climbs from the Big Lost Creek valley.

Route Details

Tennessee has more than one long trail coursing the state in addition to the fabled Appalachian Trail (AT). The Benton MacKaye Trail (BMT)—along which this hike travels—is another long-distance option. This hike is a good sampler of the BMT, which shares other parallels with the Appalachian Trail. For starters, the trail's namesake, Benton MacKaye, was the man who actually conceived the idea of an Appalachian Trail. The Benton MacKaye Trail starts at the same place as the AT, Springer Mountain in Georgia. It heads north through Georgia's Chattahoochee National Forest like the AT and intersects the AT a few times early during the 90-mile journey to the Ocoee River in Tennessee's Cherokee National Forest, not far from Chattanooga. The section in Tennessee's Cherokee National Forest is superlatively scenic as it passes through five federally designated wildernesses amid a number of rivers and mountains, including Big Lost Creek, where this hike takes place. From Cherokee National Forest, the BMT enters Great Smoky Mountains National Park near Twentymile Ranger Station. It then courses through the Smokies to terminate at Davenport Gap, on the Smokies' east end, covering a whopping 275 miles.

This section of the BMT leaves Forest Service Road 103 at an easily missed post by the road. Descend a singletrack by switchbacks, coming to Big Lost Creek at 0.2 mile. You are just a little downstream—and across the creek— from Lost Creek Campground. Join an old logging tram that runs along the left bank of the creek the entirety of the hike. Rhododendron and doghobble flank the trail, as do blasted low bluffs, created when the track was built. Beech, sycamore, and ironwood grow in the moist margins along the creek.

Benton MacKaye Trail on Big Lost Creek

By 0.5 mile, begin an elongated bend to the north and east as Big Lost Creek carves its way to meet its mother stream, the Hiwassee River. At 0.8 mile you are going fully east before you come to a hairpin bend left turn in a gorgeous area. Across the stream extends a large wooded flat where a home once stood.

You can still see remnants of rock walls along Big Lost Creek. Boring Branch comes in just downstream as the trail now heads west, entering a gorge of sorts. Here, the valley walls steepen, and Big Lost Creek caroms among big boulders, forming deep, trout-filled pools and rapids aplenty. At 1.8 miles the BMT takes you to a rock hop over Little Lost Creek entering on your left. A long pool forms around here on Big Lost Creek.

Continue descending the gorgeous vale, crossing a lesser tributary at 2.5 miles. Make one last bend to the right before reaching a trail sign at 2.8 miles. Here, the BMT leaves Big Lost Creek, climbing to join rough FS 173 en route to the Hiwassee River at Reliance. This is a good place to turn around and soak in the scenes along Big Lost Creek one more time before finishing the hike at 5.6 miles.

This hike will raise your appreciation of the BMT. Originally conceived in 1979, the Benton MacKaye Trail generally follows the western ridge of the Blue Ridge Mountains, which was the route for the Appalachian Trail as proposed by MacKaye. The BMT is a much-needed alternative to the overused Appalachian Trail for getting through North Georgia to the Smoky Mountains. It exudes a much more remote aura than the AT and is certainly less traveled.

Diamond-shaped white blazes, which signify the BMT, can be faint (not so here on Big Lost Creek). However, on the plus side, these may be the very qualities you are looking for: a challenging trail that takes effort to follow the route; a path where you must carry a lot of supplies; a trail with few over-camped spots—in other words, a trail with solitude.

Hiking the BMT is a year-round proposition, though winter is highly variable. Late spring and early summer are ideal times to hike. The BMT can become brushy and relatively buggy in late summer. Conditions improve in fall, though

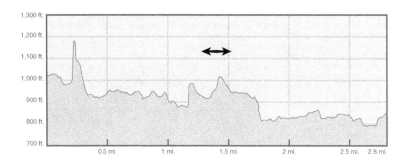

this is generally when mountain springs are at their driest. Regardless of the time of year, the BMT is nearly deserted during the week. Weekends will see a few hikers, especially around Springer Mountain, Georgia's Cohutta Wilderness, and where the BMT traverses the Smokies. If you are looking for a quality alternative long trail to the AT, the BMT is it. This hike at Big Lost Creek proves that. For trailheads, maps, driving directions, and more, visit bmta.org.

Nearby Attractions

Lost Creek Recreation Area has a 15-site campground open year-round set in a flat along Big Lost Creek, very close to this hike. Each campsite features a fire ring and picnic table. I've stayed here at least 10 nights myself. The camp has vault toilets, but you must bring your own water. In addition to hiking, visitors enjoy trout fishing in Big Lost Creek.

Directions

From Chattanooga, take I-75 north to Exit 20, and stay east with the Cleveland Bypass 6.4 miles to join US 64. Follow US 64 east 17 miles to turn left (north) onto TN 30 near Parksville Lake. Follow TN 30 north 7.2 miles to turn right onto Lost Creek Road (it becomes FS 103) and follow it 6.6 miles to the BMT, leaving left from FS 103. This spot can be hard to find. If you continue down FS 103 for 0.3 mile you will reach an alternate trailhead parking area on your right and across the bridge from Lost Creek Recreation Area.

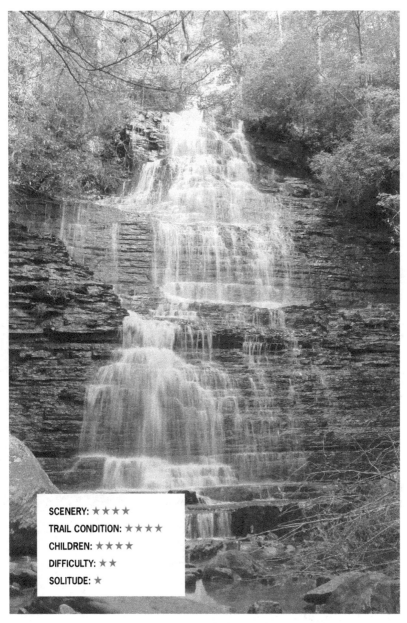

SCENERY: ★ ★ ★ ★
TRAIL CONDITION: ★ ★ ★ ★
CHILDREN: ★ ★ ★ ★
DIFFICULTY: ★ ★
SOLITUDE: ★

BENTON FALLS TUMBLES OVER 65 FEET OF LAYERED STONE.

Benton Falls

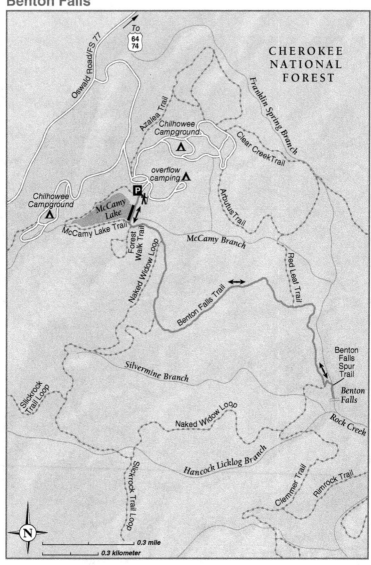

GPS TRAILHEAD COORDINATES: N35° 09.009' W84° 36.469'

DISTANCE & CONFIGURATION: 3-mile out-and-back

HIKING TIME: 2 hours

HIGHLIGHTS: Benton Falls, McCamy Lake

ELEVATION: 1,900' at trailhead, 1,690' at low point

ACCESS: Parking fee required

MAPS: National Geographic *Cherokee National Forest—Tellico & Ocoee Rivers;* USGS *Oswald Dome*

FACILITIES: Restroom, picnic tables, water, lake; swim beach, campground in season

WHEELCHAIR ACCESS: None

CONTACTS: Cherokee National Forest, Ocoee Ranger District, 423-338-3300, fs.usda.gov/cherokee

Overview

This is a popular day hike to a deservedly popular waterfall. Leave from mountaintop Chilhowee Campground, high in the Cherokee National Forest, first passing McCamy Lake. From there, take a wide path that gently descends to Rock Creek and Benton Falls. This cataract spills 65 feet into a cool, lush glen that makes for a winning destination.

Route Details

Several sidewalks in the Chilhowee day-use area converge near McCamy Lake and a large restroom. Pick up the Benton Falls Trail. Small connector trails circle the lake and also lead left to camping areas. Keep straight, crossing the dam of McCamy Lake. Look right across the mountaintop impoundment, encircled by deep forest and a trail.

Stay left on the far side of McCamy Lake, following the signs to Benton Falls. Take note of the 0.4-mile Forest Walk Trail. You can walk this loop and also circle McCamy Lake to add about a mile of hiker-only trail to your return route. For now, stay with a wide trail wandering through xeric hardwoods of oak, black

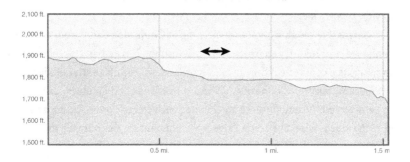

gum, sassafras, and hickory, along with a copious posse of pines. This area shows signs of past burns, giving it a brushy and ragged look. Your downgrade is moderate, and you soon leave the maze of trails around the lake. McCamy Branch, one of the primary headwaters of Rock Creek, flows to your left after leaving the lake. The other major tributary is Franklin Spring Branch. They converge unseen before forming Rock Creek and then pouring as Benton Falls.

At 0.3 mile pass the first intersection with the Naked Widow Loop, one of the many mountain bike–oriented paths in the area. Mountain bikers do use parts of the Benton Falls Trail to make loops. Ahead, the trail is often open to the sky, making it a bit warm on an August day. Walk atop open rock slabs. At 0.5 mile come to another connection with the Naked Widow Loop. Stay straight with the wide Benton Falls Trail. You are well away from Rock Creek, continuing through dry forest that seemingly leads to no waterfall.

The downgrade picks up a little, and at 1.2 miles you drift right, nearing Rock Creek. It flows to your left in lush woods that contrast with the oak forests you've been traversing. At 1.5 miles take the spur trail leading left toward Benton Falls. Descend wood, earth, and stone steps into the Rock Creek Gorge, passing near the top of the falls. Be careful—this locale has a history of accidents. Walk past stone cliffs and curve down, reaching the base of Benton Falls. Find yourself in a mossy, boulder-laden, stone-walled amphitheater ensconced in rhododendron and other evergreens, fed by the mist and flow of the falls. Above, Rock Creek spills over layered strata fanning out from its lip. When flowing well, the 65-foot falls makes a white froth, stopping only as it stair-steps downward, then slows in a boulder-bordered pool before descending to the Greasy Creek embayment of Parksville Lake below. Benton Falls are most robust from winter through early summer. In late summer and fall, the cataract can slow to a trickle.

No matter the flow rate, overnighting at Chilhowee Campground is sure to enhance your hike. Open from early April through November, this mountain-top refuge is a cool retreat during hot summer days. Popular with families who return year after year, Chilhowee fills up on weekends and holidays. Campsites can be reserved. Although there are 25 sites with electric hookups, tent camping is the norm here; the steep drive up the mountain discourages most RVs and trailers.

The campground itself spreads into three distinct areas. Loops A and B are the oldest and highest, built in the 1930s by the Civilian Conservation Corps. They are nestled in a dip on the mountain beneath a hardwood forest. A campground host keeps the area clean, safe, and secure. Loops C, D, E, and F are newer and more spacious. They are placed where the mountain terrain allows and have more ground cover for privacy beneath the piney woods.

Nearby activities include not only trails aplenty but also swimming in 3-acre McCamy Lake. At the swimming beach on the north end, sunbathers alternately lie in the sun and cool off in the water. Anglers may try to catch bream and bass from the shore, or toss a line from a small boat, as long as it's nonmotorized. As you can see, the hike to Benton Falls is just one facet of the outdoor recreation mosaic situated atop Chilhowee Mountain.

Nearby Attractions

You are near scenic and large Parksville Lake. Enjoy still-water recreation there or continue east on US 64/74 and jump on with an outfitter to tackle the wild rapids of the famed Ocoee River.

Directions

From Cleveland, take US 64/74 east 12 miles. Just past the Ocoee District Ranger Station, turn left on Oswald Road/Forest Service Road 77 for 7.3 miles. Chilhowee Campground will be on your right. Turn right toward the campground and travel 0.4 mile, passing the spur to A and B loops. Come to a fee station and the day-use area, pay your parking fee, then take the next right to reach the trailhead. There is also parking near the fee station.

27 Falls of the Scenic Spur

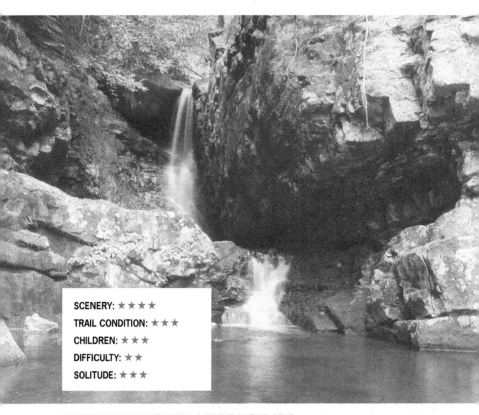

SCENERY: ★ ★ ★ ★
TRAIL CONDITION: ★ ★ ★
CHILDREN: ★ ★ ★
DIFFICULTY: ★ ★
SOLITUDE: ★ ★ ★

THE TIERED DROP OF THE FALLS OF THE SCENIC SPUR

GPS TRAILHEAD COORDINATES: N35° 06.901' W84° 34.740'

DISTANCE & CONFIGURATION: 3.2-mile out-and-back

HIKING TIME: 2.6 hours

HIGHLIGHTS: Falls of the Scenic Spur, swimming hole, Rock Creek Gorge Scenic Area

ELEVATION: 870' at trailhead, 1,180' at high point

ACCESS: No fees, permits, or passes required

MAPS: *National Geographic Cherokee National Forest—Tellico & Ocoee Rivers; USGS Caney Creek, Oswald Dome*

FACILITIES: None

WHEELCHAIR ACCESS: None

CONTACTS: Cherokee National Forest, Ocoee Ranger District, 423-338-3300, fs.usda.gov/cherokee

Overview

This hike explores the lower end of the designated Rock Creek Gorge Scenic Area in the Cherokee National Forest. Leave the trailhead to shortly enter the valley of Rock Creek, at first a wide, wooded flat centered with a clear stream. The valley closes, and you enter the heart of the gorge with its rock bluffs, boulders, and craggy splendor. A couple of creek crossings take you deeper into the gorge and trail's end, where a series of waterfalls and deep pools inspire the trail's name.

Route Details

Rock Creek Gorge is one of Cherokee National Forest's rugged and picturesque destinations. Starting atop Chilhowee Mountain, the stream flows from the greater Chilhowee Recreation Area, then carves a rock bluff–bordered chasm, littered with boulders big and small, as Rock Creek follows gravity's orders, aiming for its mother stream—Greasy Creek. You will see a concentration of falls at the trail's end. In the future, the Scenic Spur Trail may be extended up the Rock Creek Gorge, ultimately to meet Benton Falls. The heart of the gorge is also part of the 220-acre Rock Creek Gorge Scenic Area, long designated by the Cherokee National Forest as a superlatively beautiful locale.

This hike starts on the Clemmer Trail, the only path leaving the parking lot. Follow a wide track of red clay uphill and into the forest. Rock Creek is nowhere in sight and is, in fact, one watershed north of here. Ascend a small draw shaded by a white pine and tulip tree canopy. At 0.1 mile reach a trail junction. Here, the Clemmer Trail stays left and up an old roadbed, while you leave right on the Scenic Spur Trail. Work uphill through a gap, then descend another draw, now in the Rock Creek watershed. Dip into a surprisingly wide and flat valley. Hardwoods spread across this once cultivated Appalachian backwater. The hiking is as easy as the land is flat. At 0.6 mile intersect an arm of the Clemmer Trail. This arm connects the main Clemmer Trail to the Clear Creek Trail, both mountain-biking paths. This hike keeps forward under pines, sweetgum, and oaks.

At 0.9 mile Rock Creek comes into sight. The valley closes and you saddle alongside Rock Creek. Doghobble and rhododendron border pools, sandbars, shoals, and stones, as well as big boulders. It is no stretch of the imagination to see how it was named Rock Creek. At 1.1 miles the path is hemmed in by a bluff.

Falls of the Scenic Spur

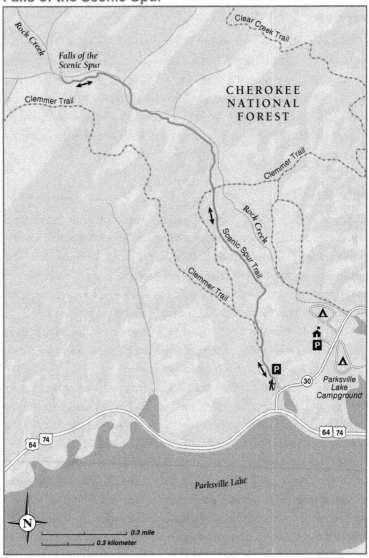

Cross over to the right bank here. In the future, the trail may be rerouted in order to avoid this crossing. At high water, expect to wet your feet, but at normal flows nimble trail trekkers can rock-hop across the watercourse. You are now on the right-hand bank, underneath birch and beech trees. The path begins ascending.

At 1.5 miles cross back over to the left-hand bank, making another rock hop. The trail is forced to the left bank by a stone bluff rising from Rock Creek. The gorge is closing tight now. The sky overhead diminishes too. Climb past a series of plunge pools divided from the trail by screens of rhododendron. As you rise farther, a rock wall surges to your left. An overhang forms a small rock house (natural rock shelter). Enter an area of more stone than vegetation and come to the set of falls. An open stone slab serves as a walkway to reach these pour-overs.

The upper fall squeezes through a cleft in a creek-wide rock rampart, briefly slowing in a long, narrow pool, shaded by overhanging rock. From there, Rock Creek pours over a second cleft into a small plunge pool. It then heads downstream about 50 feet, tumbling again into a deep pool ideal for dipping, even at summer's normally low waters. A stone bluff rises from the far side of the stream, and open waterside rock slabs and boulders make great spots for sitting and reflecting. Be aware that much of the open rock is slippery, so make all the right moves while among the rocky drops. In subfreezing weather this locale can be an icy wonderland—and as slippery as it is after a summertime thunderstorm.

Nearby Attractions

You are near scenic and large Parksville Lake. Enjoy still-water recreation there or continue east on US 64/74 and jump on with an outfitter to tackle the wild rapids of the famed Ocoee River. The trailhead is just down the road from Parksville Lake Campground too.

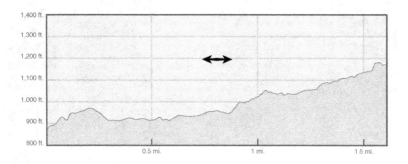

Directions

From Cleveland, take US 64/74 east 14 miles, 2.3 miles past the Ocoee District Ranger Station, to turn left on TN 30. Follow TN 30 just a short distance, then turn left onto the first gravel road and quickly reach the Clemmer/Scenic Spur Trailhead.

THE LOWER CATARACT AT TRAIL'S END FEATURES A FINE PLUNGE POOL.

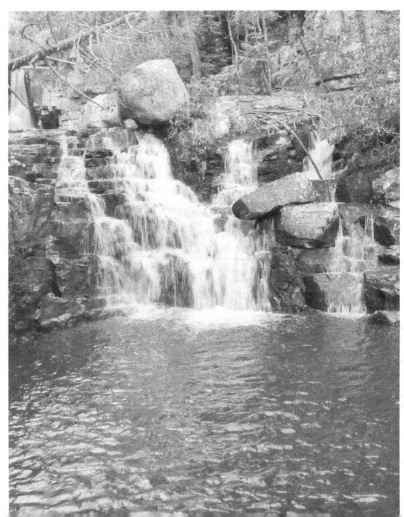

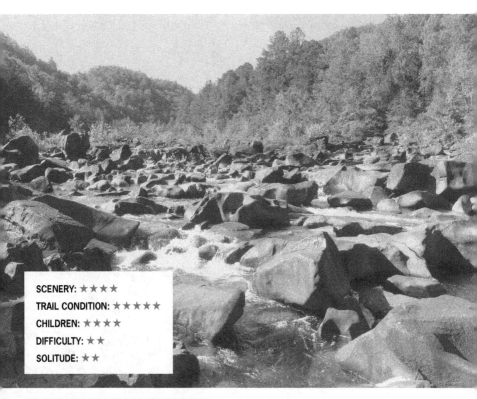

SCENERY: ★ ★ ★ ★
TRAIL CONDITION: ★ ★ ★ ★ ★
CHILDREN: ★ ★ ★ ★
DIFFICULTY: ★ ★
SOLITUDE: ★ ★

THE OCOEE RIVER CAN BE A SEA OF ROCKS.

GPS TRAILHEAD COORDINATES: N35° 03.987' W84° 27.671'

DISTANCE & CONFIGURATION: 4.8-mile out-and-back

HIKING TIME: 3 hours

HIGHLIGHTS: Ocoee Whitewater Center, historic road, Ocoee River

ELEVATION: 1,260' at trailhead, 1,390' at high point

ACCESS: Parking fee required

MAPS: National Geographic *Cherokee National Forest—Tellico & Ocoee Rivers;* USGS *Ducktown*

FACILITIES: Restroom, visitor center, store (in season)

WHEELCHAIR ACCESS: Nearby riverside trails

CONTACTS: Cherokee National Forest, Ocoee Ranger District, 423-338-3300, fs.usda.gov/cherokee

Old Copper Road Trail

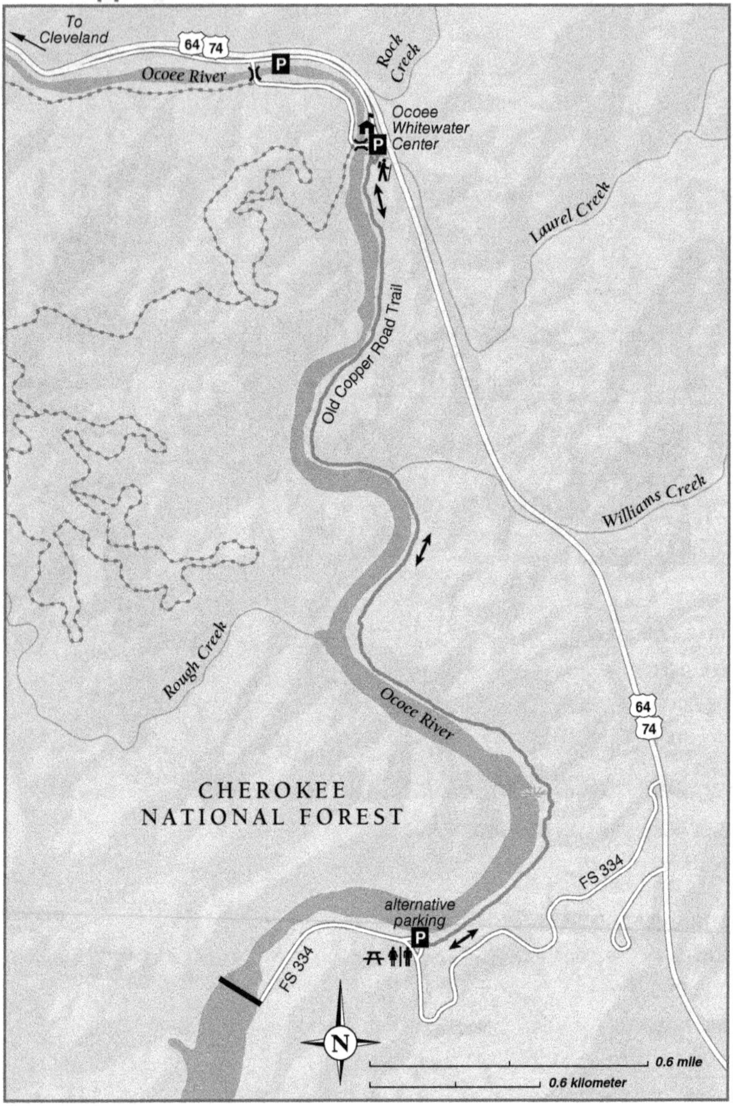

To
Cleveland
64 74
Ocoee River
Rock Creek
P
Ocoee
Whitewater
P Center
Laurel Creek
Old Copper Road Trail
Williams Creek
Rough Creek
Ocoee River
64
74
CHEROKEE
NATIONAL FOREST
FS 334
alternative
parking
P
FS 334
N
0.6 mile
0.6 kilometer

Overview

This nearly level day hike starts at the popular Ocoee Whitewater Center in the Cherokee National Forest. Trace a restored section of the Old Copper Road, once used to transport copper ore from Ducktown to a rail line in Cleveland.

Today you walk alongside the rocky Ocoee River, passing open sunning rocks and beneath wooded flats, tracing the same route of those 17 decades distant. The path is level, well marked, and easy, making it fun for anyone.

Route Details

Back in the 1830s, this remote corner of Polk County, Tennessee, was a backwater, with few people and fewer roads. Cherokee Indians still roamed the hills and hollows. This area came under US government control in the 1830s after the Treaty of New Echota. A few prospectors drifted into the Ocoee River valley, looking for gold, but instead found copper. Shipping the material was harder than mining it, with the first loads carried on the backs of mules. In 1851 work began on what is now called the Old Copper Road, a 33-mile trail linking the mines at Ducktown to a rail line in Cleveland. Ironically, much of the Old Copper Road was built by Cherokees, who remained in the region despite an effort at removal. Most of the Old Copper Road was obliterated by US 64, but the 2.4-mile stretch this trail covers faithfully follows the route of the original path over which wagons carried copper. Unbeknownst to most drivers on US 64/74 en route to the Ocoee Whitewater Center, they trace the route of the Old Copper Road.

Time moves on, and what is now the trailhead—the Ocoee Whitewater Center—was built for the 1996 Olympics and was home to the whitewater competitions for the games based in Atlanta. A whitewater paddling course was constructed near the center. Hiking and biking trails were added along the Ocoee River. A prominent footbridge crosses the Ocoee at the whitewater center. Though this hike doesn't go there, you may want to follow the all-access trail across the bridge and down the river.

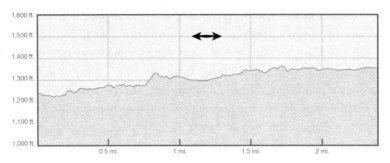

From the 30-minute courtesy parking area in front of the whitewater center, pick up a concrete trail winding downhill toward the Ocoee River. Look for a sign indicating the Old Copper Road Trail near the huge footbridge crossing the Ocoee. Come alongside the river, then immediately cross Laurel Creek on a series of flat stepping stones. The pea gravel path shortly comes to the Blue Hole, a deep river pool popular with swimmers. (By the way, water releases from the upstream Apalachia Dam can come without warning, so if you sense the river rising, head for shore.) Large sunning rocks are scattered about. The river here is dam controlled and most often has low flow, exposing an inordinate number of reddish rocks.

Keep upriver on the wide, level path shaded by shortleaf pines, holly, mountain laurel, and river birch. Briery brush can be thick in places. The path stays close to the water as the river alternates in noisy rapids and silent pools. Imagine creaky overloaded wagons pulled by sweaty horses sauntering along the very spot you walk today. Their trip from the Ducktown Basin would be hard, pulling the ore.

Spur trails lead from the Old Copper Road to rapids or smooth rock slabs. In places you can see where the trail was blasted from rock. By 0.6 mile the trail leaves the river's edge, passing through a wooded flat, straddling a hillside to your left. The river is unseen. In places the trail becomes very rooty. After climbing a little hill, cross Woods Creek on a sturdy footbridge at 1 mile. Big boulders and dense rhododendron nearly obscure the tumbling stream. Continue to follow the curves of the Ocoee River, again on a level track.

At 1.3 miles pass through another wide flat, a little distance from the river. Look for blackened trunks of trees on the uphill side of the trail. Cherokee National Forest uses prescribed fire on these pine-heavy hillsides, and the trail has been used as a fire break. Toward the river, the flat features riparian zone vegetation such as beard cane and river birch, which does not need fire to thrive.

At 1.8 miles the trail passes over an unnamed branch by culvert. At 1.9 miles bridge another unnamed stream. Just ahead, a short spur trail leaves right to a wetland and beaver habitat. An interpretive display and benches stand at the wetland edge. Beyond the wetland, the path goes over another small hill, then turns sharply with the river into a cooler, northerly exposed forest. The Old Copper Road comes back along the Ocoee, crosses one more stream, then

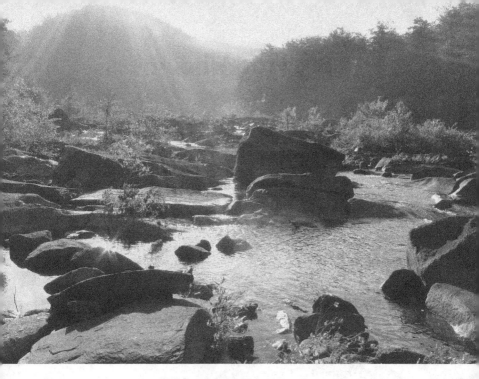

THE MORNING SUN RISES ON THE OLD COPPER ROAD.

emerges at a paddler put-in off Forest Service Road 334. This trailhead has restrooms and a picnic table, as well as parking. Since this is such a level, easy hike, it is simpler to backtrack than to arrange a one-way shuttle.

Nearby Attractions

The Ocoee Whitewater Center is a hub for paddlers, whether they are kayakers in their own boats or rafters going on a guided trip. Also, an extensive network of mountain bike trails is located across the river, using nearby Thunder Rock Campground as a jumping-off point.

Directions

From the junction of US 64 and US 64/74 Bypass, just east of Cleveland, take US 64/74 east 28 miles, 1.3 miles past Ocoee Dam #3 and Thunder Rock Campground. Reach the Ocoee Whitewater Center on your right. Enter the center grounds and park in the large lot downstream of the main building. This is fee parking.

29 Big Frog Wilderness

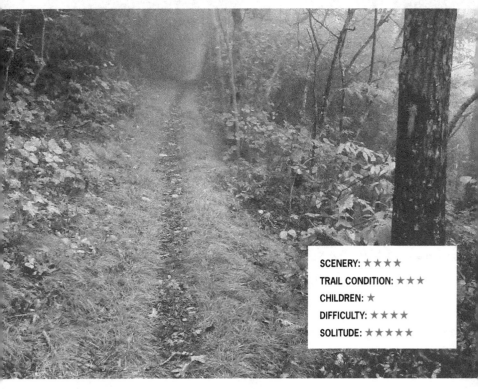

SCENERY: ★ ★ ★ ★
TRAIL CONDITION: ★ ★ ★
CHILDREN: ★
DIFFICULTY: ★ ★ ★ ★
SOLITUDE: ★ ★ ★ ★ ★

EXPECT SOME CLIMBING ON THE BIG FROG TRAIL.

GPS TRAILHEAD COORDINATES: N35° 03.278' W84° 30.067'

DISTANCE & CONFIGURATION: 11-mile out-and-back

HIKING TIME: 6.5 hours

HIGHLIGHTS: Federally designated wilderness, most western 4,000-plus-foot peak in Appalachians

ELEVATION: 2,140' at trailhead, 4,224' at high point

ACCESS: No fees or permits required

MAPS: National Geographic *Cherokee National Forest—Tellico & Ocoee Rivers;* USGS *Caney Creek, Hemp Top*

FACILITIES: None

WHEELCHAIR ACCESS: None

CONTACTS: Cherokee National Forest, Ocoee Ranger District, 423-338-3300, fs.usda.gov/cherokee

Overview

This long hike visits the Cherokee National Forest's Big Frog Wilderness. The Big Frog Trail leads from Low Gap and rises along Peavine Ridge, aiming for Big Frog Mountain. The first half of the hike is nearly level, but even after you begin climbing, the grade is moderate and steady. When the ridge narrows, outcrops afford a few views. Rise ever higher, reaching the top of Big Frog, where there is a campsite and trail intersection. The campsite is a good place to take a break before your return trip through the wilderness.

Route Details

Some hikers will climb a mountain simply because it is there. Big Frog is such a peak. Known for being the most western crag above 4,000 feet in the entire Appalachian Mountains, Big Frog and its shoulder ridges and spring branches are protected as wilderness. Most of the mountain lies within Tennessee's 8,000-plus-acre Big Frog Wilderness, but some lies within Georgia's Cohutta Wilderness, which covers a whopping 35,000-plus acres, mostly inside the Chattahoochee National Forest. Together Big Frog and Cohutta create the largest federally designated wilderness in the Southern Appalachians.

So while hiking to Big Frog you will be entirely within natural terrain, where the bears roam. Unfortunately, it is also where wild boars thrive. These exotic fast reproducers root up the land, disrupting wildflower habitat and consuming mast (fruit of forest trees) bound for native critters. I have seen boars on nearly every trip I've made into the Big Frog Wilderness. Along the way you will pass several other wilderness trails. Big Frog has an extensive trail network, with many potential loop hikes available. After this outing you will be tempted to return and create your own treks. Be apprised, the trails of Big Frog can become overgrown in summer, requiring long pants.

Leave Low Gap on the Big Frog Trail, Trail 64, passing a kiosk. Join an old woods road, heading north along the east slope of Peavine Ridge. Gently rise among white pines, oaks, and maple. In places young trees are growing up on the old roadbed, crowding the path. An easy walk leads you to the Big Frog Wilderness boundary at 0.7 mile. This preserve was established in 1984, then expanded in 1986.

Big Frog Wilderness

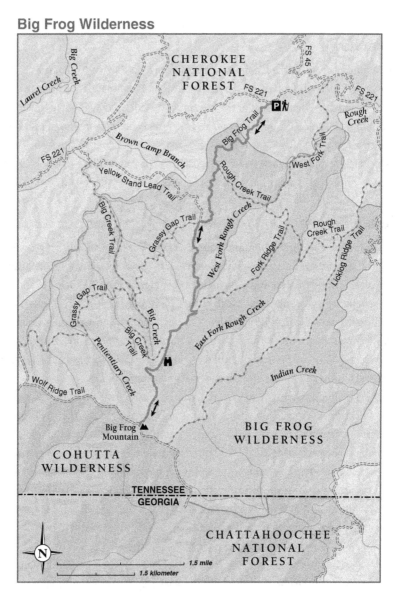

At 1.5 miles reach a trail intersection. Here the Rough Creek Trail leaves left for West Fork Rough Creek, while the Big Frog Trail keeps straight, strays from the old roadbed, and becomes a simple singletrack path hugging the slope of Peavine Ridge. Elevation changes are minimal and the climb to Big Frog

seems deceptively easy. Drift into Low Gap (same name, different place than the trailhead) at 2.3 miles, after passing through a sassafras, black gum, and pine-filled south-facing slope. You aren't much higher than when you started. Here, the Yellow Stand Lead Trail leaves right for lower Big Creek. The faint and narrow Grassy Gap Trail keeps straight for Big Creek Trail. We take the Big Frog Trail, which leaves left and begins climbing, still on Peavine Ridge.

The grade is steady but not too steep. Step over a spring branch at 2.9 miles. At 3.5 miles the trail curves around the head of a cove. Reach narrow Fork Ridge and a trail junction at 3.6 miles. Turn right here, still on the Big Frog Trail. Fork Ridge Trail leaves left. The long-distance Benton MacKaye Trail runs in conjunction with the Big Frog Trail for the remainder of the trek. Continue climbing, now on an oak ridge with a grassy understory. Partial views open east and west. The ridge becomes knife edged and rocky. Skirt around Chimneytop, then reach an easily missed trail intersection at 4.2 miles. Here, a pile of rocks, a cairn, indicates the Big Creek Trail, which leaves right down to Big Creek.

The Big Frog Trail continues to climb, wandering among rocks and trees. Reach an open vista at 4.4 miles. Here, a break in the forest allows easterly views into East Fork Rough Creek and across to Licklog Ridge. You can also look southeast to the Ocoee River basin. Curve around the point of a ridge at 4.6 miles before resuming your southbound track. The trail levels off around 4,000 feet. Enjoy some easy high-country hiking under a low canopy of wind-stunted, craggy trees.

The ridgeline widens, and at 5.4 miles the trail makes one last jump to reach the top of Big Frog Mountain and a trail junction at 5.5 miles. A level campsite is just a few steps away and makes a good spot to relax. From the

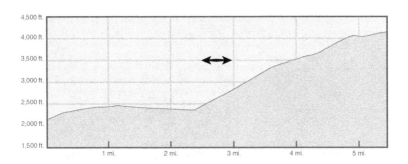

junction, the lesser-trod Wolf Ridge Trail leaves right, while the Licklog Ridge Trail heads left and downhill. A fine rocked-in spring is just 0.1 mile down the Licklog Ridge Trail. Views on Big Frog are limited by the trees, though there once was a tower up here more than a half century ago. But, you stand at the most western point above 4,000 feet in the East. Traveling across the continent you must reach western Oklahoma to once again exceed this elevation. And besides, sometimes it feels good to climb a mountain because it is there.

Nearby Attractions

The Ocoee Whitewater Center, located on US 64/74 near Thunder Rock, is a hub for paddlers, whether they are kayakers in their own boats or rafters going on a guided trip. Also, an extensive network of mountain bike trails lies across the river, using nearby Thunder Rock Campground as a jumping-off point.

Directions

From the junction of US 64 and US 64/74 Bypass, just east of Cleveland, take US 64/74 east 26 miles to the right turn at Ocoee Dam #3 and Thunder Rock Campground. Turn right and cross the dam, immediately passing Thunder Rock Campground. Join gravel Forest Service Road 45 and follow it 2.7 miles to FS 221. Turn right on FS 221 and follow it 0.7 mile to reach the trailhead parking at Low Gap on your left.

SCENES LIKE THIS ON BIG LOST CREEK BRING US BACK TO THE TRAIL TIME AND TIME AGAIN. (SEE HIKE 25, PAGE 146)

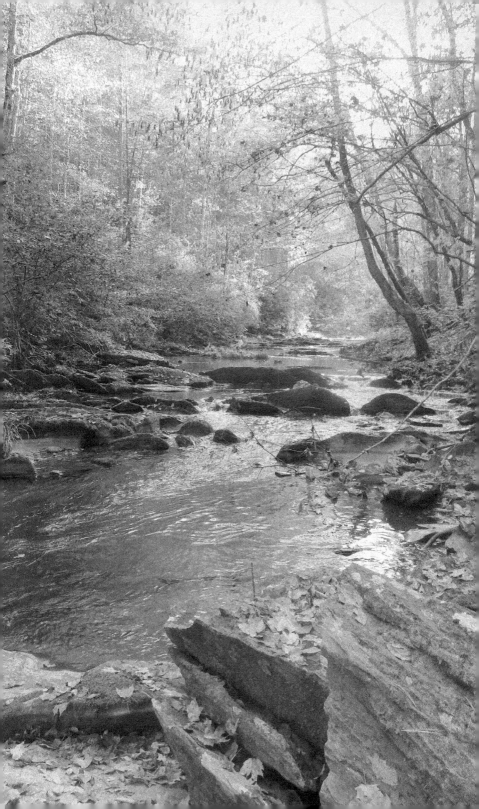

North Georgia and Northeast Alabama (Hikes 30–40)

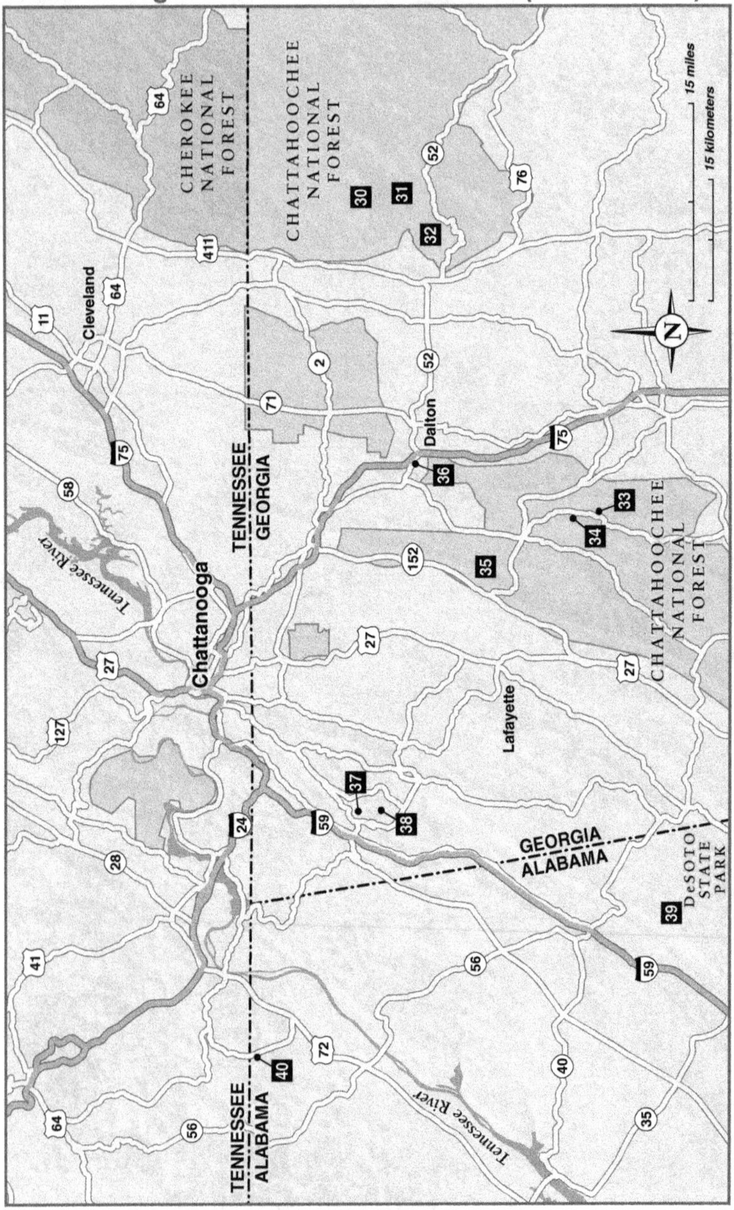

North Georgia and Northeast Alabama

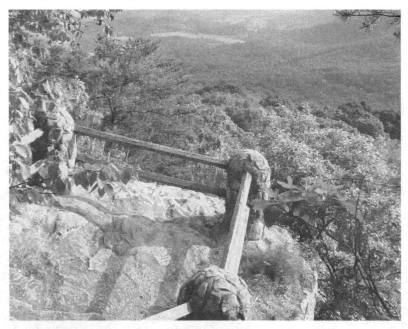

ONE OF THE MANY VISTAS YOU'LL ENJOY WHILE HIKING CLOUDLAND CANYON
(SEE HIKE 38, PAGE 214)

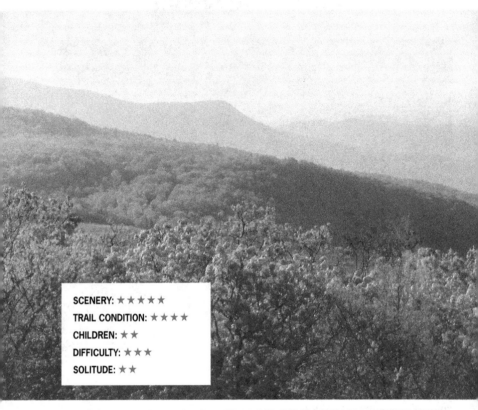

SCENERY: ★ ★ ★ ★ ★
TRAIL CONDITION: ★ ★ ★ ★
CHILDREN: ★ ★
DIFFICULTY: ★ ★ ★
SOLITUDE: ★ ★

LOOKING SOUTHEAST INTO THE COHUTTA WILDERNESS FROM GRASSY MOUNTAIN TOWER

GPS TRAILHEAD COORDINATES: N34° 51.343' W84° 39.491'

DISTANCE & CONFIGURATION: 4.4-mile balloon

HIKING TIME: 2.7 hours

HIGHLIGHTS: Tower views, mountaintop wetland

ELEVATION: 3,200' at trailhead, 3,692' at high point

ACCESS: No parking fee required at trailhead, but fee required if camping

MAPS: National Geographic *Chattahoochee National Forest—Springer & Cohutta Mountains*; USGS *Crandall*

FACILITIES: Restroom, campsites at trailhead

WHEELCHAIR ACCESS: None

CONTACTS: Chattahoochee National Forest, Conasauga Ranger District, 706-695-6736, fs.usda.gov/conf

Overview

This highland hike begins at Conasauga Lake Recreation Area, then circles a high-country beaver swamp on the interpretive Songbird Trail. From there, break off and make a moderate ascent to the peak of Grassy Mountain, where a view awaits from a metal tower.

Route Details

Be prepared to drive some gravel roads before reaching the Conasauga Lake Recreation Area Trailhead. Consider camping at Conasauga Lake to make the most of the drive. The alluring wooded locale makes for a cool summertime getaway. Want to take a dip after your hike? A ringed-off swimming beach lies across the lake from the campground. Use a canoe or small johnboat to fish for bream, bass, or trout on the 19-acre electric-motors-only lake.

The hike begins in the overflow camping area. Cross the road from the trailhead parking and pass through the campground toward campsite 3. Join the Songbird Trail, tracing old Forest Service Road 49-C, now closed and gated. Descend beneath holly and tulip trees, with uppermost rhododendron-shrouded Mill Creek to your left and young woods to your right. Interpretive signs inform hikers about managing the land for songbirds. At 0.4 mile your return route leaves left across a little footbridge. Keep straight to reach an observation deck extending into a snag-burdened beaver pond. The industrious animals have dammed Mill Creek, creating shallow ponds such as this and adding biodiversity to these mountains. Other wildlife is drawn to the wetlands, namely waterfowl.

Wooded hills frame the waters. More beaver dams downstream slow the waters of Mill Creek. Resume north on the Songbird Trail to meet the Tower Trail. It links the Songbird Trail to Lake Conasauga Campground and the 0.8-mile Lakeshore Trail, also worth your time. That path loops through evergreens around the impoundment.

Turn left on the Tower Trail, spanning Mill Creek on a bridge. Look upstream for more beaver evidence. Ascend beneath rhododendron, then climb into a more open area of shrubby woods with spicebush, mountain laurel, and blackberry. This fire-affected forest enhances songbird habitat. At 0.9 mile the Songbird Trail leaves left, and the Tower Trail splits right. Stay right with the

Grassy Mountain Tower

Tower Trail, still climbing in a thick forest. To your left, a streamlet flowing off the slopes of Grassy Mountain murmurs under thick rhododendron. The trail leaves the creek and slices through a small gap. Surprisingly, the Tower Trail briefly dips to cross a rock-strewn intermittent stream, which falls away to your right.

The climbing recommences on a rib ridge of Grassy Mountain. Pipsissewa, fern, and galax grow aplenty under pines. Make the crest of Grassy Mountain on a stony, singletrack trail. Flame azaleas color the forest orange in May. Open onto FS 49 at 1.9 miles. This road, used to access the tower, is closed to public access. The walking is easy on a smooth roadbed under an open sky. A final uptick leads to the metal structure, which you reach at 2.3 miles. The box of stubby Grassy Mountain Tower will likely be closed, but you can still climb the stairs to see past nearby wind-pruned oaks. Lands open west toward Chattanooga beyond the Conasauga River Valley below. Most of the Cohutta Mountains lie east, especially Bald Mountain and East Cowpen Mountain. Fort Mountain stands clearly in the south. Big Frog Mountain rises in the northeast. To the southeast flow waves of Georgia hills. Grassy Mountain and its tower are easily visible from US 411, traveling the Conasauga Valley below.

After climbing the tower you can easily return to the trailhead by following FS 49 downhill, but the scenery is better on the hiking trails. Therefore, backtrack 1.4 miles down the Tower Trail to the last intersection with the Songbird Trail. This time, veer right, resuming your counterclockwise circuit. Walk under rhododendron cloaking the slopes of Grassy Mountain. Cross a footbridge over a wide, rocky, low-flow branch that's more rock than water. You are now cruising along the far side of the beaver pond, and the water is visible through the forest. Bridge a second branch, then follow it downstream. Come to the lower end of the beaver swamp, bordered by rhododendron thickets and open shrubby woods. The variety of environments helps birds to thrive in this managed ecosystem. Reach upper Mill Creek at 4.2 miles. Join a footbridge to cross Mill Creek and meet a junction at 4.2 miles. You have completed the loop around the wetland. Turn right here, backtracking 0.4 mile to the trailhead.

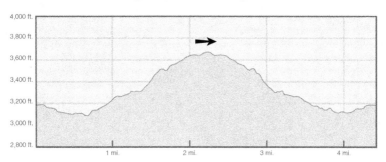

Nearby Attractions

Lake Conasauga Recreation Area has camping, swimming, and fishing during the warm season. And at 3,200 feet it will be much cooler than Chattanooga during hot spells.

Directions

From the intersection of US 411 and US 52 in Chatsworth, drive north on US 411 for 5.8 miles to Eton. Turn right on Grassy Street and follow it 0.3 mile, crossing railroad tracks to reach Crandall Ellijay Road. Turn right on Crandall Ellijay Road and follow it 0.1 mile to turn left on Mill Creek Road/FS 630. Join FS 630 for a total of 8.7 miles—the last 7.9 miles are gravel—to reach FS 17. Turn right on FS 17 and follow it 3.3 miles to reach FS 68. Turn right on FS 68 and follow it 0.3 mile, passing the right turn to Lake Conasauga Campground. Stay left with FS 49/Conasauga Lake Road. Follow FS 49 for 0.4 mile to the Lake Conasauga overflow camping area and the Songbird Trailhead. Parking is on the left side of the road.

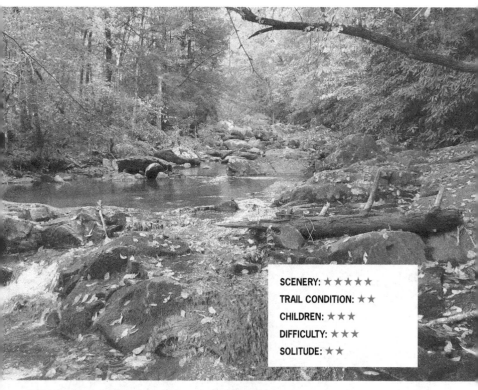

SCENERY: ★ ★ ★ ★ ★
TRAIL CONDITION: ★ ★
CHILDREN: ★ ★ ★
DIFFICULTY: ★ ★ ★
SOLITUDE: ★ ★

EMERY CREEK IS ALLURING ALL THE WAY UP TO EMERY CREEK FALLS.

GPS TRAILHEAD COORDINATES: N34° 48.737' W84° 39.102'

DISTANCE & CONFIGURATION: 4.6-mile out-and-back

HIKING TIME: 3 hours

HIGHLIGHTS: Emery Creek Falls, swimming holes

ELEVATION: 1,000' at trailhead, 1,465' at high point

ACCESS: No fees, permits, or passes required

MAPS: National Geographic *Chattahoochee National Forest—Springer & Cohutta Mountains;* USGS *Crandall*

FACILITIES: None

WHEELCHAIR ACCESS: None

CONTACTS: Chattahoochee National Forest, Conasauga Ranger District, 706-695-6763, fs.usda.gov/conf

Emery Creek Falls

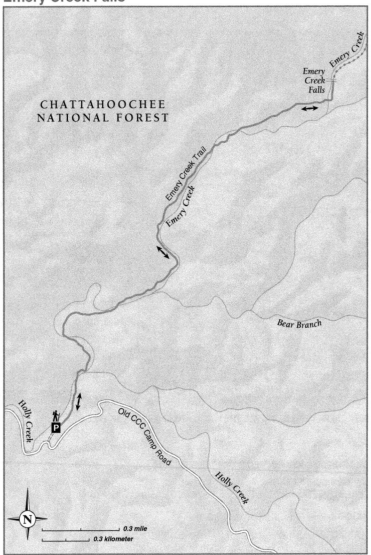

Overview

There is hardly a better way to spend a warm summer day than alongside a cool mountain stream. This particular hike starts along Holly Creek, a mountain cataract full of plunge pools ideal for swimming, with open rock slabs as excellent sunning spots too. From there, you will hike up a tributary, Emery Creek, swaddled in Southern Appalachian forest. Step over the stream numerous times to reach a gorgeous waterfall that spills in stony steps into a deep plunge pool of its own.

Route Details

This is great as a summertime family hike, or for those who just want to have fun playing in the mountains. Be apprised, the automobile-accessible swimming holes around Holly Creek can become quite crowded on warm summer weekends. Alcoholic beverages are prohibited in the Holly Creek corridor. On the hike, the several stream crossings may be challenging during winter and early spring.

Leave the parking area and clamber uphill to join an old logging grade. Holly Creek falls in big pools and noisy cascades to your left. Spur trails lead down to the clear trout-filled mountain rill. At 0.1 mile a streambed crosses the Emery Creek Trail, flowing off the steep ridge to your right. Holly Creek is now far below. Despite the extreme slope there are still a couple of user-created trails leading down to big pools. Mountain laurel, sweetgum, white pines, and chestnut oaks shade the track. By 0.2 mile you are along Holly Creek. Big boulders and open rock slabs line the crashing waterway. The depth of the pools far exceeds what you would expect for a stream of Holly Creek's size. Ahead, reach the confluence of Holly and Emery Creeks. The path is pushed to the water's edge by a steep rocky slope.

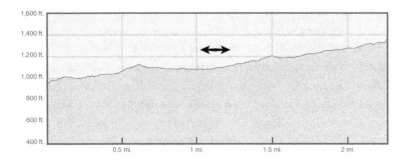

You should ford the two streams one by one. First, rock-hop or wade Holly Creek. Then you will come to a small campsite located just above the point where the two streams converge. Next, tackle Emery Creek. If you know you can't get across without getting your feet wet, consider just walking through the water. If you're going to do that, try to stay along the most level, even-bottomed section of the stream. I have seen people dangerously jump rock to rock, even though the rocks are submerged. Consider using a stout hiking stick to aid your crossing. Also, if a rock looks like it might be slippery, then it probably is, and you should certainly treat it as such. Finally, if the crossings seem too high or difficult, trust your instinct and turn back. There is no waterfall or anything on the other side that's worth risking your life for. Under normal conditions these crossings will be a simple rock hop or at worst an easy wade.

Head up the Emery Creek valley. The hillsides close in. The forest thickens. You are hiking northerly in thickets of rhododendron, doghobble, ironwood, hemlock, and black birch. Wildflowers grow rampant in this valley during spring. Cross Emery Creek again at 0.4 mile. The copious woods seem almost dark during summer. Jump over a hill as Emery Creek makes a bend. Return to Emery Creek at 0.7 mile, crossing the stream again at 0.8 mile. You are now on the left bank. Bear Branch flows in across the creek.

Cross the stream again at 1.1 miles. These are simple rock hops under normal conditions, but once you've gotten your feet wet there's no point in trying to rock-hop anymore. Just wade. You are now in a wide flat. Watch for pieces of an old jalopy, stripped of any valuable parts. It recalls images of moonshiners hauling corn liquor from stills set back in hidden, ferny hollows such as this.

At 1.3 miles cross to the left bank. The trailbed widens as you turn right and join an old woods road. The walking is easy. At 1.4 miles the old forest road crosses Emery Creek, but you stay left, resuming the singletrack footpath. Make a pair of crossings at 1.7 and 1.8 miles. The trailbed becomes quite rocky. The path and creek become separated. Return to water at 2.2 miles and cross the next stream, an unnamed tributary. Just ahead, turn left at the sign for Emery Creek Falls, tracing the now-smaller Emery Creek deeper into the mountains. Hike 0.1 mile farther to reach Emery Creek Falls. This 40-foot cascade descends in stony tiers before ending at a deep pool and an alluring swimming hole. The spur trail continues to a little hemlock flat above Emery Creek Falls and below a shorter, wider single-drop fall. Be judicious if you scramble to the upper falls.

Nearby Attractions

Holly and Emery Creeks offer not only swimming but also trout fishing. However, during warm summer weekends Holly Creek will be full of swimmers.

Directions

From Exit 336 on I-75 near Dalton, southeast of downtown Chattanooga, take US 76 east to US 411 in Chatsworth. Turn left (north) on US 411 for 2.7 miles to Eton. Turn right at the traffic light in Eton onto CCC Camp Road and follow it 7.2 miles (the road turns to gravel at 6.1 miles) to reach the trailhead on your left, just before a hard right turn.

EMERY CREEK FALLS DESCENDS IN STONY TIERS.

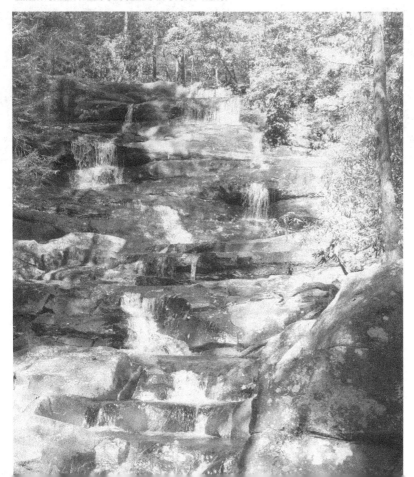

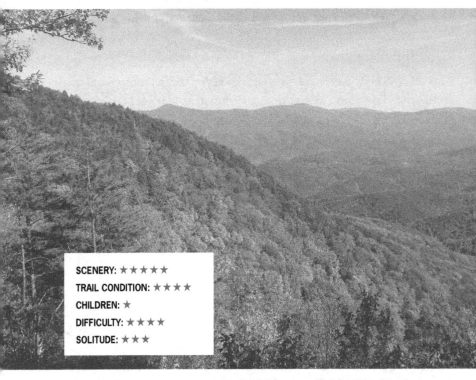

SCENERY: ★ ★ ★ ★ ★
TRAIL CONDITION: ★ ★ ★ ★
CHILDREN: ★
DIFFICULTY: ★ ★ ★ ★
SOLITUDE: ★ ★ ★

A WEALTH OF MOUNTAINS CAN BE SEEN FROM FORT MOUNTAIN STATE PARK.

GPS TRAILHEAD COORDINATES: N34° 46.730' W84° 42.321'

DISTANCE & CONFIGURATION: 7.9-mile loop

HIKING TIME: 5 hours

HIGHLIGHTS: Mountain vistas, cascades

ELEVATION: 2,730' at high point, 2,260' at low point

ACCESS: Parking pass required

MAPS: *Fort Mountain State Park Trail Map; USGS Crandall*

FACILITIES: None at trailhead

WHEELCHAIR ACCESS: None

CONTACTS: Fort Mountain State Park, 706-422-1932, gastateparks.org/FortMountain

Overview

The Gahuti Trail circumnavigates the crest of Fort Mountain, one of Georgia's most distinctive peaks, located on the western perimeter of the Cohutta Mountains. The Gahuti Trail travels through a variety of environments, from rhododendron-choked creeks to rocky overlooks to pine woods to oak forests to cool stream waterfalls. There is only a 500-foot differential between high and low elevations, but the many ups and downs aggregate to a much greater elevation change than that.

Route Details

Gahuti is Cherokee for "Mother Mountain." The Gahuti Trail is foot-traffic only, save for short stretches where bike or equestrian trails cross the Gahuti or share treadway for a brief period with the aforementioned trails. Begin your clockwise loop, following orange blazes under pines and oaks. The path parallels the main park road before joining an old roadbed at a left turn. Trace the old roadbed as it dips to a rocky hollow and then ascends it. The track becomes a narrow foot trail coursing south along the east slope of the mountain. Rhododendron, mountain laurel, and young trees crowd the path.

The path seemingly heads for every dip and hill it can find, tiring the hiker, who may complain about the ups and downs, but not about the fine scenery. Reach backcountry campsite 1, Hogpen, at 1.4 miles, just after stepping over a stream. This campsite, like the others, is merely a designated level spot with a fire ring.

The Gahuti Trail turns to bridge a bigger stream, Mill Creek, which it follows uphill, sharing trailbed with one of the park's many mountain bike trails. This is a beautiful hollow, a green cathedral of Southern Appalachia. Climb from the drainage to circle rich coves of tulip trees. Cross the main park road near the park entrance at 2.5 miles. The Gahuti Trail soon joins an old roadbed. The easy walking on this wide path under sculpted hardwoods contrasts mightily with the tangled, tight woods through which the trail passed earlier. Come to an overlook on your left at 3 miles. Cold Spring Mountain rises to the south.

Reach the spur trail to campsite 2 at 3.2 miles. The white-blazed Goldmine Creek Trail leaves right here. The upper part of Goldmine Creek is dammed,

Fort Mountain State Park Loop

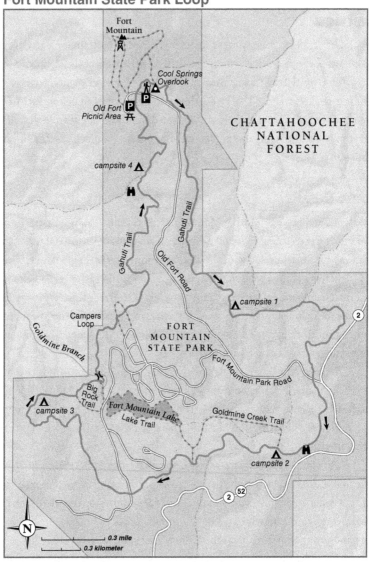

creating the 17-acre park lake, which has a swimming beach. Pass the second junction with the Goldmine Creek Trail at 3.6 miles. An extended climb follows. After leveling off, the Gahuti Trail leaves the old roadbed and winds away from the park cottages at 3.8 miles. The path becomes very rocky after crossing an old blacktop road at 4.1 miles.

The track is curving around the rocky west side of Fort Mountain. The stone-laden woods through which the path travels are among the finest in the park. Pale boulders form a backdrop against bronze pine needles, green mountain laurel, and brown tree trunks. Gain the mountain's western edge, viewing Chatsworth and the Conasauga River valley below.

Reach campsite 3, Moonshine, at 5.1 miles. This one is my personal favorite, as it is on the rim of the ridge. The view is especially alluring when the sun reflects off the ponds and lakes below, then sinks through the pine trees. Beyond the camp, the path descends to cross the first of a series of streams. The second one is bigger and is crossed via footbridge. At 5.3 miles reach a trail junction. The Gahuti Trail leaves left and the Big Rock Trail heads up and right. Partial views open through the pines before crossing the boldest stream yet, Goldmine Branch. Turn upstream, ascending beside numerous cascades, which drop in small pools before resuming their relentless whitewater-splashed reach for the valley below.

Meet the other end of the Big Rock Trail at the top of the cascades. The Gahuti crosses the stream by footbridge, then climbs to rejoin the western rim of the mountain. Pass the two ends of the white-blazed Campers Loop at 5.8 miles. Be careful at the second junction, as the Gahuti abruptly leaves left from an old roadbed. The path changes character almost instantaneously here. One minute it is on a boulder-strewn hillside pocked with pine, and the next minute it is winding along steep side slopes of a moist cove with a continuous green floor of herbs and brush.

Watch for a spur leading left in piney woods at 6.9 miles. The path drops 50 feet or so to a rock outcrop where expansive views open to the west of the

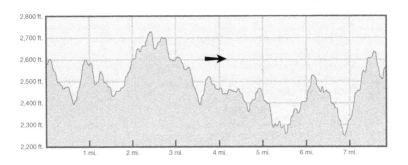

lowlands below. To the southwest is the knob of Fort Mountain where campsite 3 stands. Step over a small stream, then come to the spur for campsite 4, Rock Creek, at 7 miles. The Gahuti Trail keeps climbing along the small stream and continues in dry woods. You are ascending toward the fort part of Fort Mountain.

Cross the road to the Old Fort Picnic Area and Fort Mountain Trails at 7.6 miles. Just ahead, a spur leads left to the Fort Mountain trail network. The Gahuti turns east here, crosses a bike trail, and pops out on the Cool Springs Overlook observation deck at 7.8 miles. Holly Creek Valley lies between you and the Cohutta Mountains. Trace a paved path a short distance back to the Cool Springs parking area, completing the loop at 7.9 miles.

Nearby Attractions

Fort Mountain State Park has hiking, biking, and equestrian trails aplenty, including backcountry camping as well as a fine campground. It also has a developed campground and cottages if you are so inclined.

Directions

From Exit 336 on I-75 near Dalton, southeast of downtown Chattanooga, take US 76 east to US 411 in Chatsworth. Turn right on US 411 and follow it south a short distance to the intersection with GA 2/52, near the Murray County Courthouse. Take GA 2/52 east 7.1 miles to the state park, on your left. The Gahuti Trail starts 1.8 miles beyond the park office, at the Cool Springs Overlook parking area, on your right. Hikers using the Gahuti Trail must register at the park office before departing.

The Pocket Loop

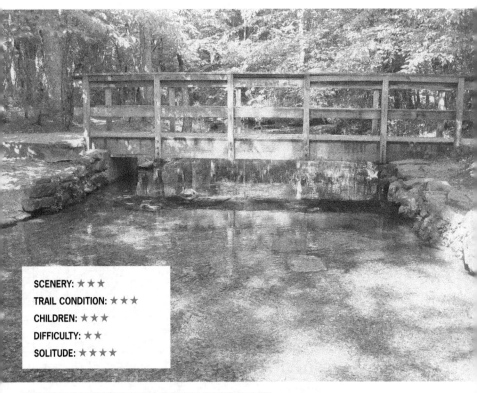

SCENERY: ★ ★ ★
TRAIL CONDITION: ★ ★ ★
CHILDREN: ★ ★ ★
DIFFICULTY: ★ ★
SOLITUDE: ★ ★ ★ ★

THIS BRIDGE SPANS THE CLEAR STREAMS OF THE POCKET.

GPS TRAILHEAD COORDINATES: N34° 35.068' W85° 04.898'

DISTANCE & CONFIGURATION: 2.8-mile loop

HIKING TIME: 1.5 hours

HIGHLIGHTS: Woodland walking, camping, spring wading

ELEVATION: 900' at trailhead, 1,000' at high point

ACCESS: No fees, permits, or passes required, unless overnighting at the Pocket Campground

MAPS: *Chattahoochee National Forest;* USGS *Sugar Valley*

FACILITIES: Restroom, picnic shelter and picnic sites, campsites near trailhead

WHEELCHAIR ACCESS: None

CONTACTS: Chattahoochee National Forest, Conasauga Ranger District, 706-695-6736, fs.usda.gov/conf

The Pocket Loop

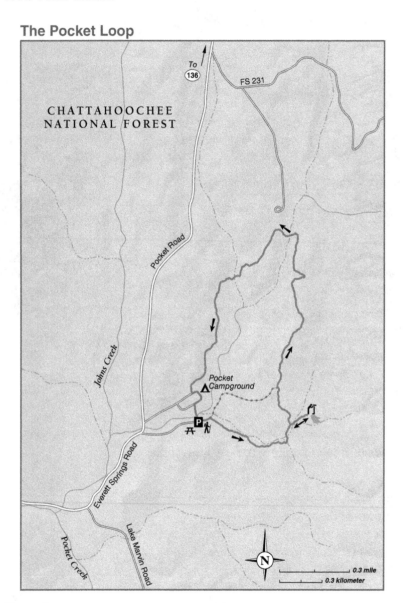

Overview

Enjoy a walk in the woods at this historic recreation area, centered by crystalline springs. Start at the alluring founts of the Pocket, then make your way up a lush hollow, eventually reaching a wildlife viewing pond. From here, the trail climbs into piney woods, circling through hills and hollows to end at the Pocket Campground. Whether it's camping or picnicking, consider adding an extra activity to your hike at this Chattahoochee National Forest recreation area.

Route Details

The Pocket is a great place to hike and camp, and it also has one of my all-time favorite Southern Appalachian names. The Pocket's location is the source of its name. Situated in the ridge-and-valley country of northwest Georgia on a large, relatively flat slice of land, a series of ridges surrounds the flat in a horseshoe shape, the flat being the "Pocket." Mill Mountain and Horn Mountain form the horseshoe. The Pocket has been a recreation destination for a long time. It started back during the Great Depression, when the Pocket housed Civilian Conservation Corps (CCC) Camp F-16 from 1938 until 1942. The CCC developed the area, as well as projects beyond the Pocket.

Today, visitors to this recreation area in the Chattahoochee National Forest can enjoy a good hike and combine it with springside camping and picnicking on Pocket Creek. Founts emit from the bed of Pocket Creek at the trailhead, ensuring year-round flow and offering yet another attraction to an already attractive locale. The springs aren't deep enough for swimming, but they do have good wading potential, especially for young hikers.

Begin the hike by passing around a pole gate. Here, the Pocket Trail leaves right. A shortcut to the main loop heads left. Stay right, heading uphill among dogwood, beech, and white pines. A spring-fed, clear stream flows to your left, forming a lush hollow. The singletrack gravel path stays above the streambed,

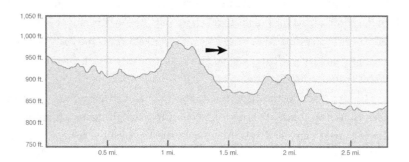

sometimes atop a low bluff. Skitter along the margin between the moist hardwoods of the stream and the drier hickories and oaks on the slope above. Interpretive signage enhances the hike. Step over the stream you have been following at 0.4 mile. Dip to cross another branch at 0.5 mile. Just ahead, a spur trail leads right. Follow this to reach a grassy wildlife clearing centered by a snag-filled pond. This pond was created for wildlife management, developing a wetland for waterfowl, beaver, and amphibians. The grasses and perimeter vegetation such as blackberries provide food for nonaquatic wildlife. Backtrack, then rejoin the loop, crossing the forest road used to develop the pond. The U.S. Forest Service might allow this closed forest road to grow back to seed.

At 0.9 mile the loop shortcut leaves left for the picnic area and campground. Keep straight here, rising into pines on a lesser-used track. Blueberries grow rife on the forest floor. The trail becomes hillier now, wandering in and out of shallow and rocky drainages broken by evergreen knolls. Note that these pine-oak woods are subject to prescribed burns in order to enhance their viability as flora, and for the sake of the attendant fauna residing within. As a result, the forest understory will be evenly aged.

The trail travels north, then suddenly turns west at 1.7 miles, dipping into the upper hollow of Pocket Creek. The stream here is likely to be dry, but a long boardwalk all but assures dry footing after heavy rains, even as you cross numerous braids of the watercourse. Reenter pine-oak woods and turn south. Dip to a second tributary at 2.1 miles, crossing this normally dry streambed sans boardwalk. Keep south, eventually descending to reach the loop road for the Pocket Campground at 2.7 miles.

This is a fine place to spend the night in the Chattahoochee National Forest. The campground road is paved, as are campsite pull-ins. A campground host is on location, caring for the neat and clean loop. Pine-oak woods tower overhead. Shade is plentiful. Some sites back up to Pocket Creek. The Pocket will fill on summer holiday weekends and on other assorted nice-weather weekends in late spring and early fall.

Getting back to the hike, follow the campground loop road left and shortly come near the developed springs area. Cross the springs on a footbridge. Since you are at hike's end, take time for a little fun with the springs. See the upwellings bubble up, adding their flow to Pocket Creek. The most reliable and

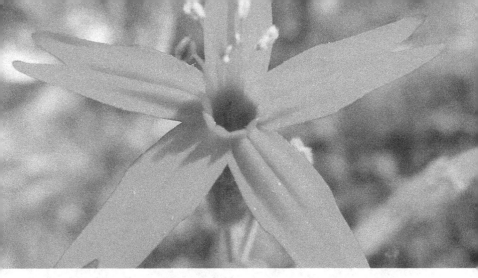

WILDFLOWERS BRIGHTEN THE TRAILSIDE FOREST.

voluminous spring is in a concrete box. The water is clear as air, and the floor of the springs is gravel, which makes it such a fine wading area. From here it's a simple stroll of a few feet to the parking area and the loop's end.

Nearby Attractions

On your way to the trailhead, you will drive part of the Ridge and Valley Scenic Byway, which essentially encircles Johns Mountain. The byway begins at GA 136 and GA 201, the route into the Pocket, then heads south on Armuchee Road to GA 27. It then heads south on GA 27, turns left on GA 156, and turns left on Floyd Springs Road to Johns Creek Road to Pocket Road. After tooling around on this marked byway, you will have a good idea of what this part of the Chattahoochee National Forest is all about.

Directions

From Exit 336 on I-75 near Dalton, southeast of downtown Chattanooga, take US 41 north/US 76 west 2.6 miles to GA 201. Turn left on GA 201 south and follow it 10 miles to the intersection with GA 136 (East Armuchee Road) at Villanow. Turn left on GA 136 and follow it 0.3 mile to Pocket Road. Turn right on Pocket Road and follow it 7 miles to the second signed left turn for the Pocket (the first is the campground entrance road; the second is the picnic area and trailhead). Drive a short distance to dead-end at the trailhead.

34 Johns Mountain Keown Falls

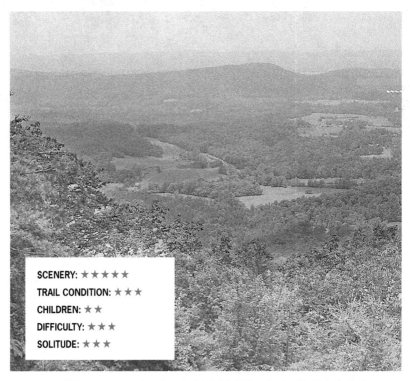

SCENERY: ★ ★ ★ ★ ★
TRAIL CONDITION: ★ ★ ★
CHILDREN: ★ ★
DIFFICULTY: ★ ★ ★
SOLITUDE: ★ ★ ★

LOOKING OUT FROM JOHNS MOUNTAIN ONTO THE RIDGE AND VALLEY PROVINCE OF NORTH GEORGIA.

GPS TRAILHEAD COORDINATES: N34° 36.810' W85° 05.293'

DISTANCE & CONFIGURATION: 4.6-mile double loop

HIKING TIME: 3 hours

HIGHLIGHTS: Keown Falls, view from Johns Mountain

ELEVATION: 1,000' at trailhead, 1,880' at high point

ACCESS: No fees, permits, or passes required

MAPS: *Chattahoochee National Forest;* USGS *Sugar Valley*

FACILITIES: Picnic area, restrooms

WHEELCHAIR ACCESS: None

CONTACTS: Chattahoochee National Forest, Conasauga Ranger District, 706-695-6736, fs.usda.gov/conf

Overview

Visit a waterfall and enjoy multiple views on this double loop. First, hike to Keown Falls (pronounced cow-an), a low-flow-but-high-drama cascade that tumbles over an undercut cliffline. From there, climb to an observation deck opening to the ridge-and-valley country of northwest Georgia. Next, cruise the crest of Johns Mountain on a level track. Return to the Keown Falls valley, making a second loop. Walk under Keown Falls to a second fall. A steady descent takes you back to the lowlands and the end of your double loop.

Route Details

Late winter and early spring are the best times to enjoy the falls and gain clear views. The rock-lined Keown Falls Trail leaves the parking area uphill. The unnamed creek of Keown Falls runs to your right—it may be bone-dry in late summer, early fall, and periods of drought. An open hardwood forest of hickory and oak greets hikers on the gentle ascent. At 0.1 mile reach the first split in the trail. Stay right toward Keown Falls. Step over the stream of Keown Falls at 0.3 mile. The hollow you are ascending narrows, then the path turns away from the hollow.

Climb onto fire-managed pine- and mountain laurel–laden south-facing slopes. Southerly views open across Johns Creek valley. Horn Mountain runs north–south. More vistas open after a switchback. The trail plies a rocky ridgeline and becomes hemmed in by a sheer stone bluff. Stone steps ease the climb. At 0.7 mile the path splits. To your left are the lower loop trail and the base of Keown Falls. Take a short walk to the falls and appreciate this 40-foot, narrow, bridal veil–type cataract. The cliffline is undercut, forming a rock house (natural rock shelter).

Backtrack from the falls and continue climbing the stone steps along the bluff. Reach a large wooden observation deck. Peer down on Keown Falls and beyond to Horn and Mill Mountains. Find the Johns Mountain Trail just a few feet ahead. Turn right here, steadily ascending an old woods road. The mountain rim drops to your right. The uppermost portion of the Keown Falls drainage flows left. Prototype pine-oak-hickory woods shade the trail. Blueberries are abundant in the understory. A short spur leads right to a partial vista before

Johns Mountain Keown Falls

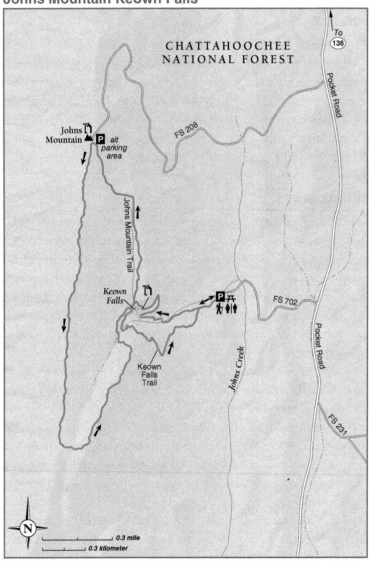

the Johns Mountain Trail turns westerly, away from the mountain edge at 1.1 miles. Reach a parking area and alternate access to the Johns Mountain Trail at 1.5 miles.

You are now 1,835 feet high, having climbed 850 feet. An observation deck overlooks the western landscape. The Armuchee Valley lies at your feet, backed by Taylor Ridge. Lookout Mountain forms the long rampart in the rear. Forest Service Road 208 has climbed Johns Mountain, the easy way for auto drivers who want to look from the observation deck.

At this point, the Johns Mountain Trail heads south, crossing grass to reenter forest. Soon pass a concrete-block structure. The trail narrows beyond the building. The woods are thick here despite the numerous boulder gardens, patterned with lichens and mosses, that dot the ridgetop. The outcrops create impromptu benches and also make good relaxation and contemplation spots. The trail is nearly level atop Johns Mountain, and the hiking easy and glorious. Broken views open through the trees, as the hillsides drop off sharply and steeply. Virginia spiderwort and fire pink wildflowers thrive among the rocks.

This part of the hike passes too fast. At 2.8 miles Johns Mountain Trail turns and comes along Johns Mountain's east rim. Partial views open east and south as you descend. Curve back into Keown Falls stream valley to cross a small creek at 3.5 miles. Ahead, a spur to the right leads to the upper edge of an unnamed fall formed by the creek you just crossed—a different fall than Keown Falls. You will soon see this fall from below. Soon come to another spur leading to an outcrop that overlooks Keown Falls. Just ahead is a low wooden bridge over the stream of Keown Falls. A few more steps end the Johns Mountain Trail and the completion of your first loop at 3.7 miles. You have been here before. Backtrack past the wooden observation deck and descend the stone stairs, returning to the base of Keown Falls.

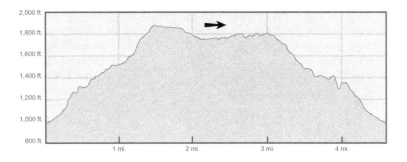

Enjoy your second helping of Keown Falls, this time continuing on the trail that passes behind and under the falls. This section is the icing on the cake—and sometimes icy in winter. Here, the pathway makes its way along the base of a dripping cliffline, where ferns and other vegetation cling to crevices. At 3.9 miles pass the second unnamed falls you saw from above earlier. This falls is about 30 feet high and a bit wider than Keown Falls. It has even less flow, however.

Descend by switchbacks away from the second falls. The hillside slope moderates as you near the lowermost trail junction at 4.5 miles. Stay right here, making the short walk back to the picnic area, finishing the hike.

Nearby Attractions

The trailhead features an attractive picnic grounds in a variety of sun and shade situations, as well as a restroom. Consider bringing a picnic. The nearby Pocket Recreation Area, also part of the Chattahoochee National Forest, offers a picnic area of its own, along with a high-quality campground.

Directions

From Exit 336 on I-75 near Dalton, southeast of downtown Chattanooga, take US 41 north/US 76 west 2.6 miles to GA 201. Turn left on GA 201 south and follow it 10 miles to the intersection with GA 136 (East Armuchee Road) at Villanow. Turn left on GA 136 and follow it 0.3 mile to Pocket Road. Turn right on Pocket Road and follow it 4.9 miles to the signed right turn for Keown Falls Recreation Area and FS 702. Turn right on FS 702 and follow it 0.6 mile to dead-end at the trailhead.

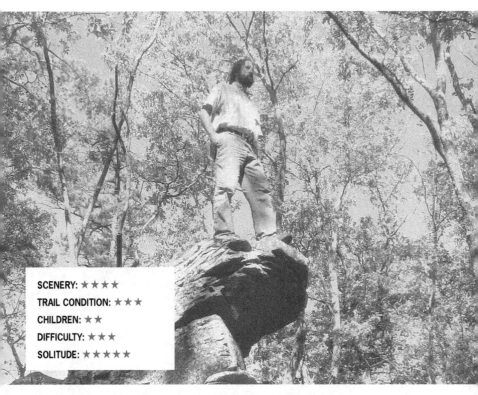

SCENERY: ★ ★ ★ ★
TRAIL CONDITION: ★ ★ ★
CHILDREN: ★ ★
DIFFICULTY: ★ ★ ★
SOLITUDE: ★ ★ ★ ★ ★

THE AUTHOR STANDS ON AN OUTCROP FOUND AT MILE 3.1 OF THIS HIKE.

GPS TRAILHEAD COORDINATES: N34° 36.810' W85° 05.293'

DISTANCE & CONFIGURATION: 6.2-mile loop

HIKING TIME: 4 hours

HIGHLIGHTS: Solitude, mountain creeks

ELEVATION: 1,020' at trailhead, 1,610' at high point

ACCESS: No fees, permits, or passes required

MAPS: *Chattahoochee National Forest;* USGS *Catlett*

FACILITIES: None

WHEELCHAIR ACCESS: None

CONTACTS: Chattahoochee National Forest, Conasauga Ranger District, 706-695-6736, fs.usda.gov/conf

Dicks Ridge Circuit

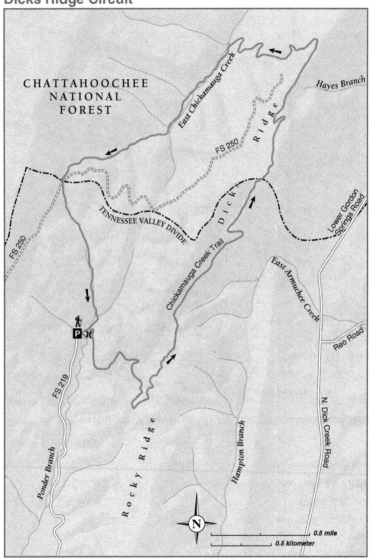

Overview

This hike rewards hikers with solitude amid rich bottomland forests and craggy ridgetop woodlands. Start on clear Ponder Branch, then meander north and climb Dicks Ridge, zigzagging on old roadbeds and singletrack paths before descending to East Chickamauga Creek. This stream displays quiet subtle beauty and a remote feel, as the trail heads up the intimate valley, shaded by stately beech trees. A final climb leads back into the Ponder Branch watershed, where many creek crossings take you downhill to your point of origin.

Route Details

The Chickamauga Creek Trail is not immediately evident. Look to the right-hand side of the lowermost metal gate for the path. Pick up the lightly trod Chickamauga Creek Trail to cross Ponder Branch on a wooden footbridge. Turn upstream, briefly tracing Ponder Branch. Turn right here, away from the power line clearing. Begin working the steep ridge slope. The leveled footbed winds in and out of dry stream drainages. Look for evidence of a fire from years past— blackened bases of tree trunks and even aged brush on the forest floor. Parts of this loop will weave in and out of former burns. Fire is important for the health and staying power of pine-oak-hickory forests, which thrive on the ridgelines of northwest Georgia. Periodic fires keep these woodlands open, enrich the soils for the surviving trees, and prevent alteration of the ecosystem by the introduction of less fire-tolerant species. See if you can spot the former burn areas.

Climb to reach a gap at 0.9 mile. The path switchbacks up the ridgeline in oaks. Reach a power line clearing at 1.5 miles. Blackberry bushes will be full of ripe fruit in midsummer along the clearing. Cross the power line clearing and reenter woodland, angling right, still on a narrow footpath, still in a northeasterly direction.

Views can be had off to the east, depending on weather and foliage. At 2 miles turn left, joining an old roadbed. Steadily ascend onto Dicks Ridge, only

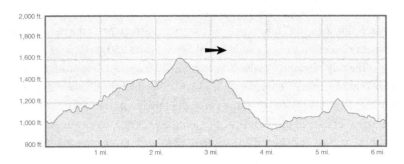

to turn back right, still climbing. The walking becomes an easy woods stroll atop the crest of the ridge. But just as you are getting comfortable the Chickamauga Creek Trail unexpectedly splits left off the ridgecrest at 2.6 miles and becomes singletrack. Be aware, as a game/hunter trail keeps forward. The trail is marked with white blazes throughout its length and also has brown plastic Carsonite posts at confusing places.

The trail once again becomes a footpath and descends in loping switchbacks, then levels off amid an extremely rocky area. Look for an unusual rock formation at 3.1 miles. Here, a conspicuous rock rises upward at its base, then has an outward diving board–like extension on top. It seems a perfect place for a politician to make a speech to his rocky constituents. Leave left off the ridge not far past the unusual rock and join another old roadbed, which continues a downward trend. At 3.6 miles the old logging road splits. Stay downhill and to the right, ever winding toward the flats of Chickamauga Creek, which are reached at 4.1 miles.

This branch is actually East Chickamauga Creek. It flows north to meet West Chickamauga Creek and leads to the famed Civil War battlefield of the same name. Soon step over a couple of feeder branches of Chickamauga Creek, then cross the creek itself at 4.4 miles. This small, shallow, crystalline stream gurgles gently over rocks and makes for a dry crossing in times of normal flow. Continue up the slender valley bordered by steep hillsides, broken only by feeder branches that form their own tight hollows. Birdsong echoes in this intimate valley that exudes a wild aura.

Creekside beech trees are abundant. These moisture-loving giants with the smooth gray bark show off leaves of gold in the fall. In spring, dwarf crested iris, a delicate purple-and-white wildflower, brightens the bottomlands. Step over East Chickamauga Creek three more times. By this point, the watercourse is barely flowing and all feeder branches are intermittent. After the last crossing the path rises steeply to a gap and Forest Service Road 250 at 5.3 miles.

The ridge dividing Ponder Branch from Chickamauga Creek forms part of what is known as the Tennessee Valley Divide. North of the divide, water flows into the Tennessee River, then the Ohio, the Mississippi, and into the Gulf in Louisiana. Ponder Branch, south of the Tennessee Divide, flows into Armuchee Creek, then into the Oostanaula River to the Coosa River, then the Alabama River, which flows into the Gulf at Mobile Bay.

The Chickamauga Creek Trail crosses FS 250 at an angle and reenters the woods about 150 feet beyond where it emerged. It is all downhill from here. Step over Ponder Branch six times before crossing a feeder branch and opening onto a power line clearing. Cross the clearing, join a roadbed, and reach the trailhead, finishing the hike.

Nearby Attractions

Hikers can also enjoy primitive car camping along FS 219 near the trailhead.

Directions

From Exit 345 on I-75 near Ringgold, Georgia, southeast of downtown Chattanooga, take US 41/76 south 0.4 mile to Bandy Road. Turn right onto Bandy Road. At 5 miles Bandy Road becomes Old Ringgold Road. Keep straight here and follow it 4.6 more miles to reach GA 201. Stay right here, joining GA 201 and continue south 5.7 miles to reach GA 136 in Villanow. Turn right on GA 136 (East Armuchee Road) and follow it 4 miles to Ponder Creek Road. Turn right onto Ponder Creek Road and follow it 0.6 mile to FS 219. Veer right onto FS 219 and follow it 1.7 miles to dead-end at the trailhead parking area.

ASTERS ADD COLOR TO THE SCENERY ON THIS HIKE.

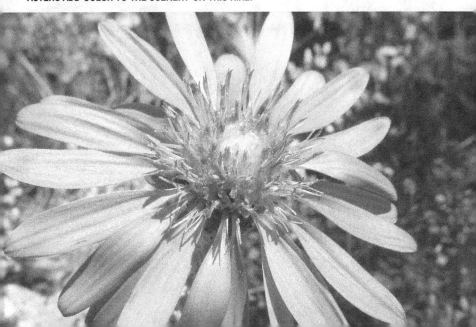

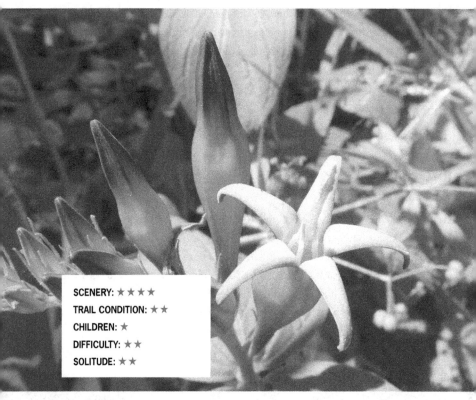

SCENERY: ★ ★ ★ ★
TRAIL CONDITION: ★ ★
CHILDREN: ★
DIFFICULTY: ★ ★
SOLITUDE: ★ ★

INDIAN PINK IS A SHOWY SUMMERTIME FLOWER FOUND ALONG THE GEORGE DISNEY TRAIL.

GPS TRAILHEAD COORDINATES: N34° 47.912' W85° 00.692'

DISTANCE & CONFIGURATION: 1.4-mile out-and-back

HIKING TIME: 1.5 hours

HIGHLIGHTS: Open vistas from rock face

ELEVATION: 840' at trailhead, 1,525' at high point

ACCESS: No fees, permits, or passes required

MAPS: *George Disney Trail*; USGS *Tunnel Hill*

FACILITIES: None

WHEELCHAIR ACCESS: None

CONTACTS: City of Dalton, Georgia, 706-278-5404, cityofdalton-ga.gov

Overview

This short-but-tough hike scrambles up the north side of Rocky Face Mountain, climbing to the grave of a Confederate soldier en route to far-ranging views from open outcrops that give this peak its name. Since it isn't far to the top from the trailhead, anybody can make the climb, taking ample breaks. A fit person can make it without stopping.

Route Details

When people hear the term Disney Trail, they don't think of hiking near Dalton, Georgia. But in fact there exists a fine path that leads to a spectacular view. According to the historical marker at Mill Creek Gap, just below the trailhead at the Georgia State Patrol headquarters, a wild volley from Union forces during the Battle of Rocky Face killed one George Disney. This Confederate soldier, who immigrated to Kentucky from England, was part of a human telegraph chain roughly following the trail up Rocky Face Mountain, keeping Confederate forces apprised of Union troop movements from the open rock outcrops, the same one you will hike to 16 decades later. And it is a stellar view. Of course, the panorama we enjoy for aesthetic reasons was, to George Disney, a strategic Civil War military post in much the same way as was Chattanooga's Lookout Mountain.

The trailhead is atypical and your first time driving to it will seem a little strange. But yes, you do drive directly up the steep driveway of the Church of the Nazarene. The trail's beginning is clearly marked. Join a singletrack dirt path overlain upon an old faded roadbed. A rich hardwood forest grows tightly, and the understory brush will be thick during summertime. This trail has a well-deserved reputation for steepness, but at this point the path is only gently climbing, and you can't help but wonder when the real ascent begins.

After you become used to the pleasant nature of the path, it suddenly turns left from the old roadbed and scrambles up the north side of Rocky Face Mountain. This north-south–running ridge was wracked by storms in June 2011. You will still find downed trunks around which the trail was rerouted. Despite this rerouting, the path travels mostly straight up the mountain, sometimes slipping between standing rocks and boulders. This north-facing slope harbors a surprising number of spring wildflowers, including Indian pink. This

George Disney Trail

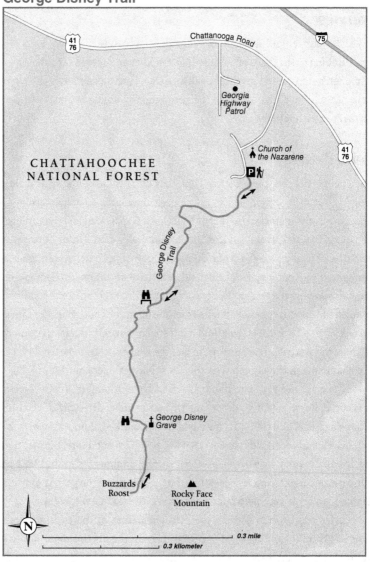

deep red tubular flower with a yellow tip grows on shady slopes such as this and also along streambeds. North Georgia is near the center of its range.

At 0.4 mile come to a bench. This was placed here by Boy Scouts, who generally maintain this trail. You will thank them for this bench, and it is well used, given the steepness of the path. Partial views open from past storms. You can see the parallel lanes of I-75 streaming to and from Chattanooga, as well as Rocky Face Mountain north of Mill Creek Gap. Over time, this view will once again close as the forest rises from the fallen hardwoods rotting back into the soil. Most likely you will be simply trying to catch your breath, rather than contemplating views or forest renewal. The time comes to recommence climbing, and the path winds ever more among rocks, around the fallen trunks, and always up.

At 0.5 mile the ridge becomes rockier. Westerly views open, framed in shortleaf pines. And it keeps getting better. By 0.6 mile you have reached an open outcrop to the right of the trail. Here, you have unimpeded views of East Chickamauga Creek Valley below and a series of north-south–running ridges beyond. These views will pale in comparison only to the panoramas that lie ahead. But first, as you continue up the trail, reach the grave of George Disney. This burial place was rediscovered by local Boy Scouts while on a hike in 1912. They found the rocky internment adorned with a simple pine board. This they replaced with the marble marker you see today. Of course, that marker is now more than a century old. Disney's grave remains a somber site, a reminder of the cost of war.

Continuing, work a little higher up the mountain to reach the Buzzards Roost at 0.7 mile. Here, a wide-open outcrop presents panoramas as far as the eye can see. This was the locale of Confederate scouts watching the movements of Union troops below during the 1864 Battle of Rocky Face, when Confederate General Johnston was vainly trying to stop William Sherman's infamous March to the Sea, where he laid waste to Georgia. Rather than pass through Mill Creek Gap, Sherman outflanked Johnston, and Rocky Face Mountain was abandoned. But for George Disney, a bullet ended his life on this rocky ridge.

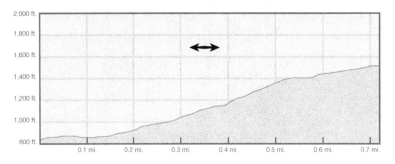

Here at Buzzards Roost, Scouts have built a wooden outdoor amphitheater with seats. Still, most people repose on the open rocks with the fantastic views. On a clear day you can see Lookout Mountain, Signal Mountain, and points between here and there. Interestingly, if you drive Georgia 201 south from the town of Rocky Face, these outcrops are easily visible. From Buzzards Roost, an old dirt road leaves the mountain and a faint trail keeps south on Rocky Face. Plans are in the works to route the long-distance Pinhoti Trail along the crest of Rocky Face Mountain.

Nearby Attractions

Other recreation destinations, located in the Chattahoochee National Forest—namely the Pocket, Keown Falls, and the Ridge and Valley Scenic Byway—are south of here.

Directions

From Exit 336 on I-75 near Dalton, southeast of downtown Chattanooga, take US 76 west/US 41 north 0.7 mile, then turn left up the steep driveway into the First Church of the Nazarene. Pass the main church building on your left to hit a T intersection, then make a left and go just a short distance to the trailhead, within close proximity to the Tipton Life Center building. The path is marked with a sign.

Sitton Gulch Trail

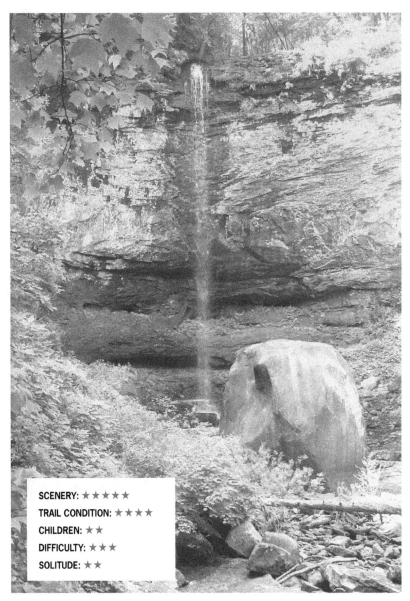

SCENERY: ★ ★ ★ ★ ★
TRAIL CONDITION: ★ ★ ★ ★
CHILDREN: ★ ★
DIFFICULTY: ★ ★ ★
SOLITUDE: ★ ★

CHEROKEE FALLS IS A REWARDING DESTINATION.

Sitton Gulch Trail

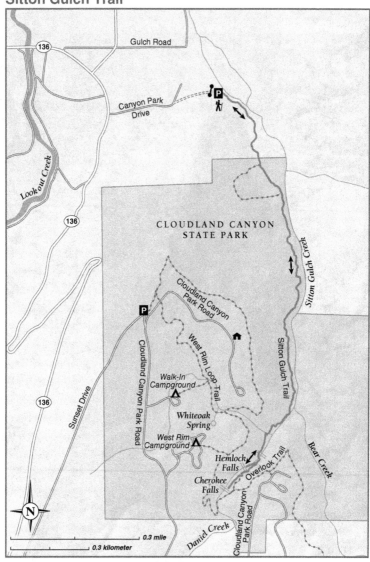

GPS TRAILHEAD COORDINATES: N34° 51.595' W85° 29.078'

DISTANCE & CONFIGURATION: 4.8-mile out-and-back

HIKING TIME: 3.5 hours

HIGHLIGHTS: Three waterfalls, boulder-strewn canyon

210

ELEVATION: 820' at trailhead, 1,570' at high point

ACCESS: Entrance fee required

MAPS: *Cloudland Canyon State Park Trails;* USGS *Durham*

FACILITIES: Restrooms at trailhead

WHEELCHAIR ACCESS: None

CONTACTS: Cloudland Canyon State Park, 706-657-4050, gastateparks.org/cloudlandcanyon

Overview

This hike explores the inner reaches of the Sitton Gulch, traveling into the heart of this rock-walled, boulder-filled watery canyon. Despite the extremely rugged terrain, the well-constructed path makes its way along Sitton Gulch Creek before turning into the tighter gorge of Daniel Creek. Here, the hike culminates in a visit to three impressive consecutive waterfalls. It's a steady climb to the cascades but well worth the trip. You will be rewarded with an easy return hike back to the trailhead.

Route Details

Leave the shady parking area to walk around a pole gate. Begin walking south into Sitton Gulch. At this point the canyon is quite wide, and Sitton Gulch Creek is normally just a rocky streambed split into braids off to your left. By the way, the valley that is Cloudland Canyon was known only as Sitton Gulch until 1939, when the state of Georgia began acquiring the land for a state park. I can only surmise that the tourism marketing department thought Cloudland Canyon sounded more alluring than Sitton Gulch. Name notwithstanding, the valley is a natural wonder, carved by eons of water flowing off Lookout Mountain. There

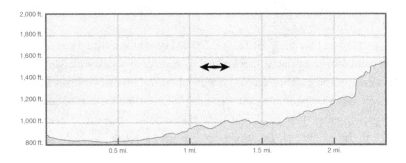

have been geological events here too. Hundreds of boulders have tumbled from clifflines above, forming obstacles to the gorge's waters.

You will likely hear no water flowing at the hike's beginning. Here, Sitton Gulch Creek flows underground, only occasionally filling the adjacent streambed. The wide trail leads through a mostly level valley under verdant hardwoods of sugar maple, white oak, shagbark hickory, and beech, along with a few shortleaf pines. Ferns and wildflowers thicken in spring. Pass a pair of spurs making a loop to your right at 0.4 and 0.6 mile. Soon you will come along a flowing part of Sitton Gulch Creek, working its way among gigantic boulders of every shape and size. The gorge is closing and the trail is rising.

Between the forest, stream, and geology it's easy to see why Sitton Gulch was a perfect choice for a Georgia state park. Rock bluffs reach for the sky. Tulip trees soar straight and regal, lording over big pools where the waters of Sitton Gulch Creek have stilled. At times the trail is forced away from the water, working around big boulders or rock fields. The user-friendly path, about 3 feet wide and lightly graveled, makes the walking incredibly easy considering the irregular nature of the valley bottom.

At 1.7 miles you can look down at the confluence of Bear and Daniel Creeks, which come together to form Sitton Gulch Creek. The trail turns up the valley of Daniel Creek. The hollow noticeably narrows, and the valley walls steepen. At 1.9 miles cross the rocky wash of Whiteoak Spring. The gorge is bordered with sheer clifflines, rubble fields, and incredibly large boulders. At 2 miles the Sitton Gulch Trail comes alongside an unnamed waterfall. This cataract spills over a big protruding ledge into a plunge pool backed by a stone bluff across the creek. Hemlocks and hardwoods are motionless spectators, watching the water drop. From here, the path steepens, then crosses a bridge to reach the left bank of Daniel Creek. Make sure and look back at the unnamed falls from this bridge.

Intersect the spur to Hemlock Falls just beyond the bridge. Turn right here and tread deeper up Daniel Creek, skirting the edge of a rock wall. Reach Hemlock Falls and an observation platform at 2.1 miles. This cascade spills about 60 feet off a rock ledge, landing with a mighty splash. Note the pair of monstrous old-growth tulip trees growing astride the waterfall observation deck. Backtrack to the bridge over Daniel Creek. To reach Cherokee Falls, take the steep stone steps, which lead to a set of staircases that will simply amaze. Level decks between staircases allow hikers to catch their breath. The time and effort to build these steps is something to contemplate. However, also ponder the incredibly steep slope that would otherwise be impassable if not for the steps.

At 2.3 miles intersect the connector leading up to the West Rim Loop Trail and the main park access to the waterfalls. Most people take the short way from the main park access atop Lookout Mountain to the falls or otherwise make the circuit of the West Rim Loop Trail (detailed in Hike 38). Return to Daniel Creek, reaching Cherokee Falls at 2.4 miles. From your rocky perch you can look across at a wide and deep plunge pool into which a white ribbon spills 70 feet over a sheer stone face, encircled by an echoing amphitheater of rock and vegetation. This is an ample reward for your climb, but as you return down the gorge, take time to admire the beauty that may have been overlooked on your arduous trek up Sitton Gulch.

Nearby Attractions

Cloudland Canyon State Park offers multiple hiking trails, tent camping, trailer camping, and cabins.

Directions

From Exit 11 on I-59 southwest of Chattanooga, take GA 136 east 1.5 miles to Canyon Park Drive, marked by a pair of stone gates. Turn left and follow Canyon Park Drive past houses 0.5 mile to turn right into the Cloudland Canyon State Park, Sitton Gulch access.

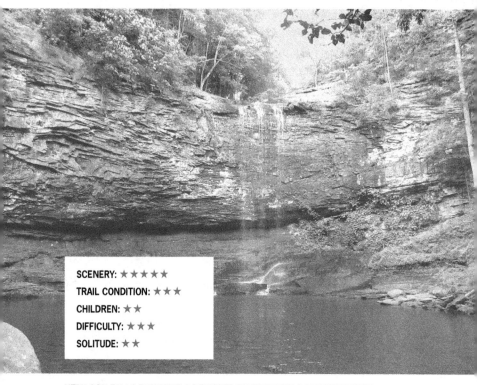

SCENERY: ★ ★ ★ ★ ★
TRAIL CONDITION: ★ ★ ★
CHILDREN: ★ ★
DIFFICULTY: ★ ★ ★
SOLITUDE: ★ ★

HEMLOCK FALLS FASHIONS A DELICATE CURTAIN WHILE DROPPING INTO
A LARGE PLUNGE POOL.

GPS TRAILHEAD COORDINATES: N34° 50.081' W85° 28.831'

DISTANCE & CONFIGURATION: 5-mile loop

HIKING TIME: 3.5 hours

HIGHLIGHTS: Multiple canyon views, Cherokee Falls

ELEVATION: 1,700' at trailhead, 1,940' at high point

ACCESS: Entrance fee required

MAPS: Cloudland Canyon State Park Trails; USGS Durham

FACILITIES: Restrooms, picnic areas at trailhead

WHEELCHAIR ACCESS: None

CONTACTS: Cloudland Canyon State Park, 706-657-4050, gastateparks.org/cloudlandcanyon

Overview

The rewards exceed your efforts on this highlight reel of a hike. Grab an initial valley view from the trailhead, then dip into the lushly wooded, waterfall-rich canyon of Sitton Gulch. Bridge Daniel Creek and begin a loop. Cruise upland hardwoods, then take in a far-reaching northward vista. Turn into the west rim of Sitton Gulch, where more overlooks from sandstone slabs inspire.

Route Details

Be prepared to take plenty of photos and videos on this trek. Join a paved path at the canyon edge heading left, but you will soon stop to admire stellar panoramas of layered sandstone alternating with greenery seen beyond the safety rails in the chasm below. The pavement soon gives way to dirt and gravel, as the yellow-blazed West Rim Loop Trail passes behind park rental cabins. Soon, the noise of Daniel Creek crashing through Sitton Gulch drifts to your ears.

The path is wide, rocky and rooty, and heavily traveled here. Head deeper into Sitton Gulch. Pines, oaks, mountain laurel, and rhododendron border the trail. At 0.3 mile reach the spur to Cherokee and Hemlock Falls. The canyon is exceedingly steep here, thus the park has built elaborate stairways leading into the canyon depths. This stairwell dips along the sheer bluff, then divides. Take the spur to Cherokee Falls, negotiating step after step to reach the falls base. The huge plunge pool is backed by a semicircular rock cathedral over which Cherokee Falls spills in a white ribbon. To reach Hemlock Falls, take the steps and decks astride the unstable canyon walls.

After returning from the falls on stairs galore, catch a breath, descending toward Daniel Creek into a mass of mountain laurel and rhododendron. The waterway is much calmer here compared to the falls below, snaking between rock slabs and gathering in little pools to your right. Cross Daniel Creek by footbridge at 0.7 mile. Climb from Daniel Creek on a series of switchbacks. Unfortunately, other hikers have chosen to shortcut these switchbacks, creating a maze of trails. Stay with the yellow blazes and you will be okay. Remember, no official trail travels directly up or down a mountain slope. The user-created trails not only add confusion but also lead to erosion and watershed siltation.

Cloudland Canyon Vistas

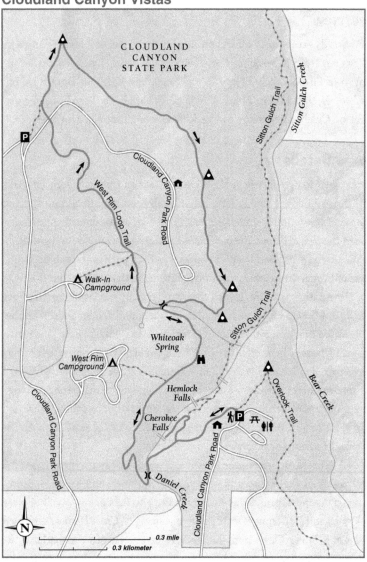

Watch for a little trailside cave on a switchback. A few hikers have ridden out a thunderstorm in that cubbyhole. Regain the canyon rim amid oaks and pines. At 1.2 miles meet a spur leading left to the West Rim Campground. Keep straight on the West Rim Loop Trail, tracing the painted blazes. Come alongside wide rock slabs, broken by slender but deep clefts over which you step. Reach a particularly wide rock slab at 1.3 miles that reaches to the edge of the rim and offers vistas into the upper canyon. Peer into the deep crevasses dividing the biggest slabs. The West Rim Loop Trail follows the canyon edge, where brushy vegetation persists on thin rocky soils, and wooden safety rails guard the most precarious locations. Partial views continue into Sitton Gulch.

The West Rim Loop Trail leaves Sitton Gulch and turns into the stream of Whiteoak Spring, cutting its own minicanyon. Come alongside the spring and reach the loop portion of the hike at 1.5 miles. To your right, across a small wooden bridge, is your return route. Stay left and continue up the trickling stream of Whiteoak Spring, in its own shallow valley. At 1.8 miles pass the spur trail to the walk-in tent camping area, then step over what remains of Whiteoak Spring. Pines increase in number as the trail gently lifts. Walk among exposed rock slabs well away from the canyon rim before crossing a park-cabin access road at 2.3 miles. At the edge of the mountain a short spur leads left to a parking area, but stay right, heading north along the rim edge. The town of Trenton and the Lookout Creek Valley are visible through the trees.

The West Rim Loop Trail levels off, weaving through Table Mountain pines broken by gray boulders. Thorn-laden blackberry bushes crowd the trail in summer, where tree cover is sparse. Reach the hike's most northerly point and a spur to a fantastic overlook at 2.6 miles. Stroll down to a projecting rock and feast your eyes on the yonder. Lookout Creek and the Tennessee River Valley are flanked by rising wooded ridges. The west brow of Lookout Mountain stretches toward the horizon.

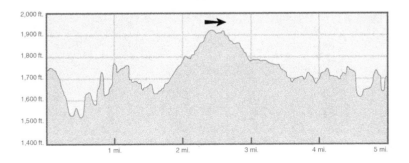

The West Rim Loop Trail turns south from here, skirting Sitton Gulch. Blueberry bushes carpet the woodland floor. Ahead, numerous marked spur trails link the West Rim Loop Trail and more park cottages. Stay with the yellow blazes. Other spur trails lead left to small outcrops, some providing more of a vista than others. Sitton Gulch narrows as you head deeper into the canyon. The rock walls of the far rim become closer and their size and color impresses. Pass an overlook at 3.2 miles and another developed one at 3.5 miles. Here, you can see Bear Creek cutting its own gorge to meet Daniel Creek to form Sitton Gulch Creek. The next developed overlook delivers a view across the canyon to the picnic area where this hike begins. Look for the grassy lawn and wooden safety rails. Falls and rapids are clearly audible below at this overlook. From here, the path turns away from the main gorge and travels the bluffline of a small mini-canyon created by Whiteoak Spring. Reach the stream responsible for this land-form at a wooden bridge at 3.8 miles. You have been here before, and the loop portion of the hike is complete. Backtrack to Daniel Creek and its bridge, then ascend to reach the picnic area at 5 miles.

Nearby Attractions

Cloudland Canyon State Park offers multiple hiking trails, tent camping, trailer camping, and cabins.

Directions

From Exit 11 on I-59 southwest of Chattanooga, take GA 136 east 8 miles to the state park. Once in the state park, follow Cloudland Canyon Park Road straight to near its end at 1.5 miles, near the scenic overlooks.

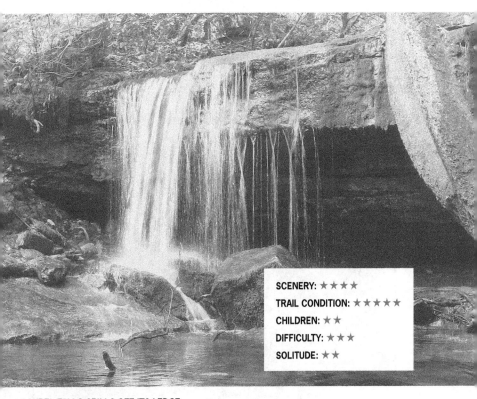

SCENERY: ★ ★ ★ ★	
TRAIL CONDITION: ★ ★ ★ ★ ★	
CHILDREN: ★ ★	
DIFFICULTY: ★ ★ ★	
SOLITUDE: ★ ★	

LAUREL FALLS SPILLS OFF ITS LEDGE.

GPS TRAILHEAD COORDINATES: N34° 30.085' W85° 37.130'

DISTANCE & CONFIGURATION: 5.5-mile loop

HIKING TIME: 3 hours

HIGHLIGHTS: Geological formations, waterfalls, history

ELEVATION: 1,480' at trailhead, 1,760' at high point

ACCESS: No fees, permits, or passes required

MAPS: DeSoto State Park; USGS Valley Head, Dugout, Fort Payne, Jamestown

FACILITIES: Camp store, nature center, restrooms, picnic area, campground

WHEELCHAIR ACCESS: None

CONTACTS: DeSoto State Park, 256-845-0051, alapark.com/parks/desoto-state-park

DeSoto State Park Loop

Overview

This loop cobbles a multitude of trails to form a "highlight reel" of Alabama's DeSoto State Park. First, the Quarry Trail snakes among boulders and other rock formations to reach a Civilian Conservation Corps (CCC) pit used in developing the park in the 1930s. Join the serpentine Family Bike Loop, then enter the striking Laurel Creek Valley, walking over open stone slabs and beside big boulders framed in mountain laurel, rhododendron, and azaleas. Visit three waterfalls: Lost Falls, Laurel Falls, and Azalea Cascades. Explore an amazing boulder garden, then finish the loop.

Route Details

The Quarry Trail Trailhead isn't obvious. As you are looking out the Country Store's front porch, walk left toward the campground access road. The white-blazed Quarry Trail starts on the far side of the campground access road. The singletrack path, also open to mountain bikers, enters pine-oak-holly woods on a trailbed of rocks, roots, and needles. Meander along a hillside gently ascending to reach a boulder garden at 0.4 mile. Giant graybacks are strewn along a hill, and the Quarry Trail takes you between them, sometimes dividing and taking diverse routes that rejoin. Watch for rock overhangs among the boulders.

Dispersed boulders continue to flank the path as you circle a cove at 0.9 mile. The trail itself is not particularly rocky, however. Reach the CCC quarry pit at 1 mile. Here an interpretive sign explains the mission of the New Deal public works agency. Cut blocks lying in the quarry stand as unfinished relics of young men's work. DeSoto State Park opened in 1939. Today, the quarry resembles an ancient abandoned amphitheater. Briefly pick up an old roadbed, likely used to haul the quarry blocks. A backcountry campsite access trail leaves right, but you split left then and quickly leave the roadbed. Climb a bit and reach the primitive campground access road and the high point of the loop, nearly 1,760 feet, at 1.4 miles.

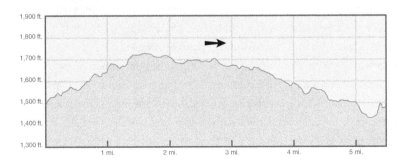

The Quarry Trail rambles into a grove of shortleaf pines to reach an intersection at 1.7 miles. Here, the Family Bike Loop begins its torturous 1.9-mile convolution through scrub pines, fields, and woods. Take it for the additional trail mileage, as it is very easy and mostly level. The meandering path travels past an old water tower at 2 miles and in every cardinal direction before reaching the Lost Falls Trailhead. You can avoid the Family Bike Loop by keeping straight at this junction and then turning left on the silver-blazed Campground Trail, which reaches the Lost Falls Trailhead much more directly.

Arrive at the Lost Falls Trailhead and a paved road at 3.6 miles. Keep straight, crossing the road to pick up the hiker-only Orange Trail, as it passes a rock inscribed with trail mileages. The Never Neverland Trail leaves right, making a separate mountain bike loop. The Campground Trail leaves left to the park campground. The Orange Trail heads south, often traveling over open rock slabs and under pines. Step over a clear tributary at 3.8 miles. At 4 miles reach a trail junction in an open rock flat. The Blue Trail leaves south to cross Laurel Creek (the Blue Trail doesn't access Laurel Falls). Stay left with the Orange Trail as it heads down to Laurel Creek as well, to reach Lost Falls at 4.2 miles. A spur loop leads right to the actual drop. The two-tiered aquatic surge spills over a curved stone ledge. Note the rock overhang on the north bank.

Keep downstream along tumbling Laurel Creek, flanked by pockets of mountain laurel and rhododendron. The trail turns away from the watercourse as it circles into tributary watersheds, wandering atop copious deer moss–ringed rock slabs bordered by shortleaf pines, holly, and oaks. At 4.5 miles a spur leads left to the campground. At 4.8 miles another spur leads right downhill to Laurel Falls. At this cascade, the creek flows over a horizontal rock rampart, splashing onto a rock pile, then settling down in a clear, calm pool.

The loop continues in alluring Laurel Creek Valley. Step over a tributary just before reaching a junction at 5 miles. Here, another spur leads left to the campground. Stay with the Orange Trail, and note the climbing boulder—popular with kids—to the right. Now, the hike enters a nest of interconnected trails used by park visitors who want just a short stroll. Bridges span Laurel Creek. Azalea Cascades is a small falls that spills over a rock slab after sneaking under some gigantic boulders. It is reached at 5.3 miles. The bridge below Azalea Cascades has a wide observation deck over Laurel Creek. The deck is part of the Azalea Boardwalk, an

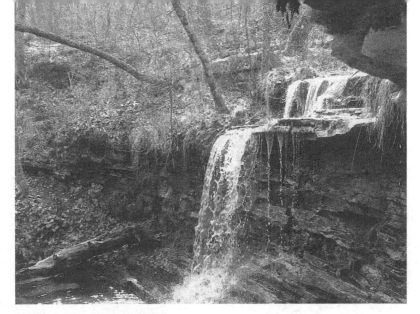

LOST FALLS MAKES ITS DOUBLE DROP.

all-access trail. Finally, head north through a crazy cluster of colossal boulders, including Needle Rock. Pick your route, aim for the Country Store, and you will have completed your loop.

Nearby Attractions

DeSoto State Park has a host of attractions. First, you can camp in a tent or RV, stay in a cabin or chalet, or check in to a full-service lodge. It also has a restaurant, golf course, and more, in addition to the trails and other natural aspects of this Lookout Mountain getaway.

Directions

From Exit 231 on I-59, southwest of Chattanooga, take AL 117 south 5.7 miles, passing through Hammondville and Valley Head to reach the town of Mentone. Turn right on County Road 89 and follow it 5.8 miles, then turn left at an intersection, still on CR 89. Travel for 0.5 mile, then turn right again at another intersection, still on CR 89. Continue 0.4 mile to reach the right turn into the Country Store at DeSoto State Park. Park here, toward the campground access road. The turns aren't as confusing as they sound, since they are all signed for DeSoto State Park.

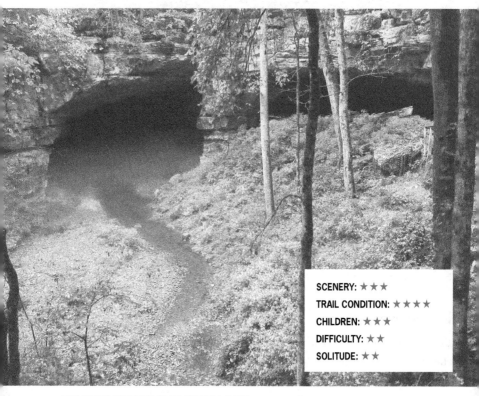

SCENERY: ★ ★ ★
TRAIL CONDITION: ★ ★ ★ ★
CHILDREN: ★ ★ ★
DIFFICULTY: ★ ★
SOLITUDE: ★ ★

DRY CREEK EMERGES FROM RUSSELL CAVE.

GPS TRAILHEAD COORDINATES: N34° 58.723' W85° 48.585'
DISTANCE & CONFIGURATION: 1.5-mile loop with spur
HIKING TIME: 1 hour
HIGHLIGHTS: Historic cave, museum
ELEVATION: 660' at trailhead, 1,060' at high point
ACCESS: No fees, permits, or passes required
MAPS: *Russell Cave National Monument;* USGS *Doran Cove*
FACILITIES: Restrooms, water, museum at trailhead
WHEELCHAIR ACCESS: Between visitor center and Russell Cave
CONTACTS: Russell Cave National Monument, 256-495-2672, nps.gov/ruca

Overview

Learn about a historic rock shelter and cave while on this shorter trek. First, take an all-access path to the mouth of Russell Cave and an adjoining rock shelter, home to American Indians for 10,000 years. Then make a loop on a steep but paved path along the east slope of Montague Mountain. Explore rocky woods while learning interpretive information about the life of the hunters and gatherers who roamed these hills. *Note:* The cave grounds are open 8 a.m.–4:30 p.m. Central Time. The monument gates are locked at 4:30 p.m.

Route Details

Russell Cave National Monument is an undervisited resource of the National Park Service in the greater Chattanooga area. The 310-acre site hosts a visitor center, picnic area, and hiking trails, all centered around an incredible cave and rock shelter utilized by aboriginals for thousands of years until the mid-1600s. It is generally regarded as the oldest continuously inhabited rock shelter in the eastern United States.

And after you visit, you'll see that the setting is ideal for a shelter. The rock overhang is quite large and was created after part of Russell Cave collapsed, closing access to the netherworld. However, just next to it, the cave is open. And from the maw flows Dry Creek, providing water access for shelter inhabitants, whether they be residents, winter residents, or hunters just passing through.

Jackson County, Alabama, home of Russell Cave, is said to have more underground passages than any other county in the United States. The underground system of this mountainous area is a labyrinth of dark waterways—an underground plumbing system, if you will. Interestingly, the flows of Dry Creek rise and fall with the rains that make their way through the greater Chattanooga area. So when you visit the cave, Dry Creek may live up to its name, or it may flow furiously.

Take some time to explore the visitor center, "boning up" on the archaeological history of Russell Cave. You can see the actual tools used by the prehistoric residents. Also, grab a trail map while you are there. As you face the visitor center, head left toward a gazebo and the beginning of the all-access trail to Russell Cave. Join an elevated boardwalk, heading south along the slope of Montague Mountain, which rises to your right. A stony, hardwood forest of ash,

Russell Cave National Monument

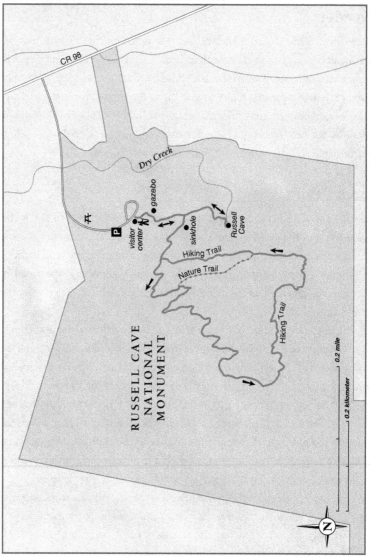

dogwood, and oak shades the path. An open field brightens the flats beyond the trail. Shortly, pass the intersection with the simply named Hiking Trail. Continue straight, aiming for Russell Cave. After a quarter mile you will curve into a hollow created by Dry Creek. Turn the corner and enter a dramatic setting.

Here, the open mouth of Russell Cave lies at the base of a cliffline, emanating water. Fog, sometimes present due to the different air temperatures inside and outside the cave, may hang around the mouth. To your right the historic arched rock shelter forms a twin opening in the rock face. Continue along the board-walk, overlooking the gravel bars of Dry Creek, until you are at the shelter.

Full-size mannequins replicate aboriginals at work and play in the cave. Interpretive information enhances the experience. Take note that ranger-led cave tours are held daily at 11 a.m. Central Time. Take a few minutes to absorb the atmosphere, then backtrack to the Hiking Trail, arriving at 0.3 mile.

On the Hiking Trail, you will first pass a large sinkhole, part of Jackson County's underground plumbing system. Head uphill on a narrow, paved track. Stay right as the path splits in a loop. This east slope of Montague Mountain is very rocky but forested with red cedar, shagbark hickory, and chestnut oak, which grow wherever they can find soil. Wind uphill using switchbacks. Enjoy interpretive information scattered alongside the path.

At 0.5 mile the natural-surface Nature Trail leaves left and shortcuts the loop. Stay with the Hiking Trail, twisting through boulder gardens, land so rocky as to thin the forest. Continue loping up the mountainside, passing occasional resting benches perfect for those surprised by the continuous ascent. Watch for smaller sinkholes scattered among the rocks and trees in this karst terrain. The Hiking Trail levels off at 0.8 mile. Congratulations, you just climbed 400 feet!

It isn't long, though, before you begin to lose the hard-won elevation. The descent uses switchbacks as well. Watch your footing if the path is wet, especially in steep sections. Level off before meeting the other end of the Nature Trail at 1.2 miles. Continue along mid-slope, completing the Hiking Trail loop

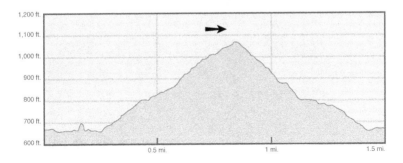

at 1.3 miles. From here it is a simple backtrack to the visitor center. You may be tempted to visit Russell Cave one more time on your return trip.

Nearby Attractions

Russell Cave National Monument offers visitors a shaded picnic area.

Directions

From Chattanooga, take I-24 west toward Nashville, to Exit 152A, west of the split with I-59. Follow US 72 west toward Scottsboro, Alabama, and at 8.5 miles turn right on two-lane Jackson County Road 75 north. Follow CR 75 for 1 mile, then turn right on CR 98. Follow CR 98 for 3.7 miles, then turn left into the monument. Follow the monument entrance road to the visitor center.

DO YOU HEAR THE TRAIL CALLING YOU?

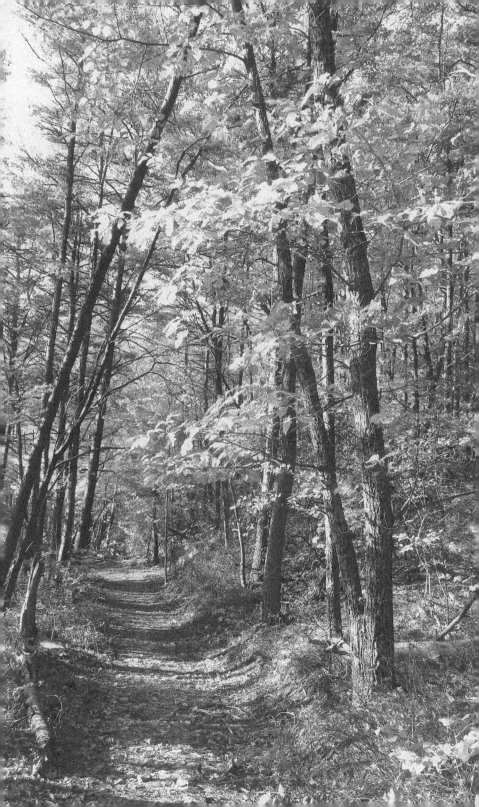

Appendix A:
Outdoor Retailers

ROCK/CREEK NORTH SHORE

301 Manufacturers Road

Chattanooga, TN 37405

facebook.com/rockcreekoutfitters

ROCK/CREEK HAMILTON CROSSING

2200 Hamilton Place Blvd.

Chattanooga, TN 37421

423-485-8775

facebook.com/rockcreekoutfitters

They also have locations in Riverside, as well as downtown Chattanooga and in Cleveland and on the Ocoee.

DICK'S SPORTING GOODS

Hamilton Place Mall

2100 Hamilton Place Blvd., Suite 102

Chattanooga, TN 37421

423-535-9584

dickssportinggoods.com

Appendix B: Hiking Clubs

OUTDOOR CLUB SOUTH—CHATTANOOGA CHAPTER

meetup.com/Chattanooga-Outdoor-Club-South

OUTDOOR CHATTANOOGA

423-643-6888

outdoorchattanooga.com

CHATTANOOGA HIKING CLUB

chatthiking.com

CHATTANOOGA HIKING MEETUP

meetup.com/Chattanooga-Hiking-Meetup

Index

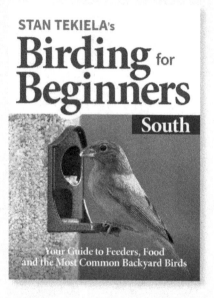

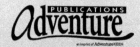

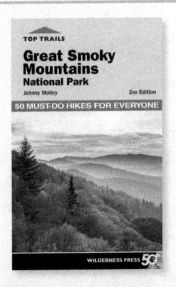

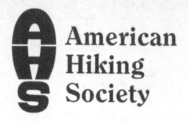

American Hiking Society

PROTECT THE PLACES YOU LOVE TO HIKE.

Become a member today and
take $5 off using the code **Hike5**.

AmericanHiking.org/join

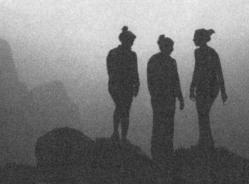

American Hiking Society is the only
national nonprofit organization dedicated
to empowering all to enjoy, share, and
preserve the hiking experience.

About the Author

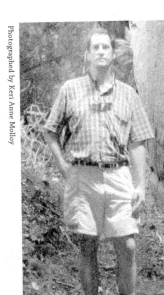

JOHNNY MOLLOY is a writer and adventurer, based in East Tennessee, who has lived in the shadow of the mountains for more than three decades. His outdoor passion started on a backpacking trip in Great Smoky Mountains National Park with Chattanooga native Calvin Milam. That first foray unleashed a love of the outdoors that has led to his spending countless nights backpacking, canoe camping, and tent camping for the past 30 years. Friends enjoyed his outdoor adventure stories; one even suggested he write a book. He soon parlayed his love of the outdoors into an occupation. The results of his efforts are more than 75 books. His writings include hiking, camping, and paddling guidebooks; comprehensive guidebooks about a specific area; and true outdoor adventure books. Molloy has also written numerous articles for magazines, websites, and newspapers. He continues writing and traveling extensively throughout the United States, endeavoring in a variety of outdoor pursuits. His other interests include serving God as a Gideon, studying American history, and following University of Tennessee sports. For the latest on Johnny, please visit johnnymolloy.com.

DEAR CUSTOMERS AND FRIENDS,

SUPPORTING YOUR INTEREST IN OUTDOOR ADVENTUR
travel, and an active lifestyle is central to our operations, fro
the authors we choose to the locations we detail to the way w
design our books. Menasha Ridge Press was incorporated in 198
by a group of veteran outdoorsmen and professional outfitters. F
many years now, we've specialized in creating books that benefit tl
outdoors enthusiast.

Almost immediately, Menasha Ridge Press earned a reputatio
for revolutionizing outdoors- and travel-guidebook publishin
For such activities as canoeing, kayaking, hiking, backpackin
and mountain biking, we established new standards of qualit
that transformed the whole genre, resulting in outdoor-recreatio
guides of great sophistication and solid content. Menasha Ridg
Press continues to be outdoor publishing's greatest innovator.

The folks at Menasha Ridge Press are as at home on a whitewate
river or mountain trail as they are editing a manuscript. The books w
build for you are the best they can be, because we're responding t
your needs. Plus, we use and depend on them ourselves.

We look forward to seeing you on the river or the trail. If you'd lik
to contact us directly, visit us at menasharidge.com. We thank you fo
your interest in our books and the natural world around us all.

SAFE TRAVELS,

Bob Sehlinger

BOB SEHLINGER
PUBLISHER

CPSIA information can be obtained
at www.ICGtesting.com
Printed in the USA
JSHW040818220920
8125JS00002B/2